DIET AND NUTRION FOR BEGINNERS

THIS BOOK INCLUDES :

" THE CARNIVORE DIET AND AIR FRYER COOKBOOK"

BY DAVID CLARK

Air Fryer Cookbook

100 Quick, Easy and Delicious Affordable

The trademarks that are used are without any consent, and the publication of the trademark is without permission or backing by the trademark owner. All trademarks and brands within this book are for clarifying purposes only and are owned by the owners themselves, not affiliated with this document.

Introduction

Air fryers use dry air and less oil to cook your food. As per an estimation, 40 calories are found per teaspoon of oil (120 calories per tablespoon). The small amount of fat you add makes the results all too delicious and extra crispy to brown and caramelize. The amount you can see in the air fryer is basically nothing compared to the amount of oil in deep-fried foods, contributing to fewer calories than the normal fried food when saturated fat. The benefits of using an air freezer actually outweigh the risks. Besides that, the food turns out crispy and crunchy.

Air Fryer Recipes

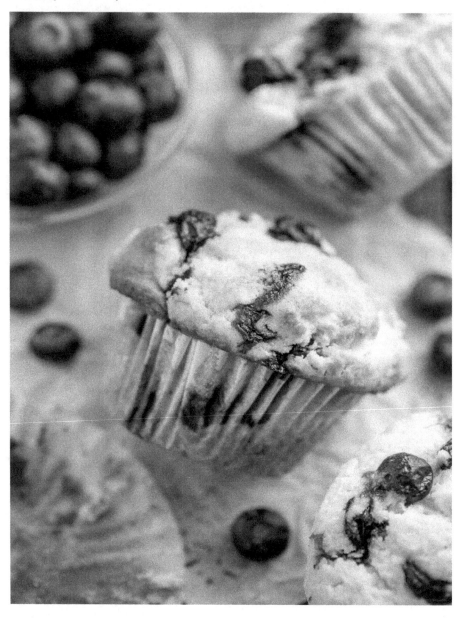

1.Squash Oat Muffins

Total time: 30 min

Prep time: 10 min

Cook time: 20 min

Yield: 12 servings

Ingredients:

- Two eggs
- 1 tbsp. pumpkin pie spice
- 2 tsp. baking powder
- 1 cup oats
- 1 cup all-purpose flour
- 1 tsp. vanilla
- 1/3 cup olive oil
- 1/2 cup yogurt
- 1/2 cup maple syrup
- 1 cup butternut squash puree
- 1/2 tsp. sea salt

Directions:

1. Strip 12 cups of a cupcake muffin tin with liners.

2. Wire rack insertion at rack position 6. Pick bake, set temperature to 390 f, 20-minute timer. To preheat the oven, press start.

3. Whisk together the milk, vanilla, oil, yogurt, maple syrup, and squash puree in a large bowl.

4. Mix together the rice, pumpkin pie spice, baking powder, oatmeal and salt in a shallow dish.

5. Apply the mixture of flour to the mixture and whisk to blend.

6. Scoop the batter and bake it for 20 minutes in a prepared muffin tin.

7. Enjoy and serve.

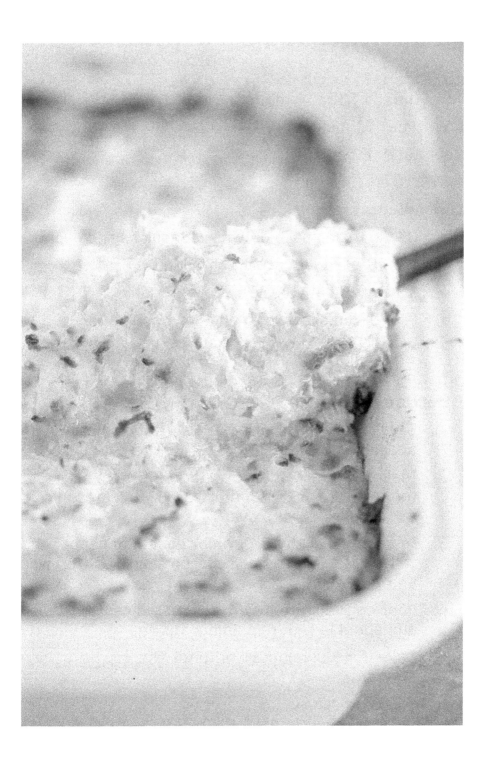

2.Hash brown Casserole

Total time: 1 hour 10 min

Prep time: 10 minutes

Cook time: 60 minutes

Yield: 10 servings

Ingredients:

- 32 oz. frozen hash browns with onions and peppers
- 2 cups cheddar cheese, shredded
- 15 eggs, lightly beaten
- Five bacon slices, cooked and chopped
- Pepper
- Salt

Directions:

1. Spray 9*13-inch casserole dish with cooking spray and set aside.
2. Insert wire rack in rack position 6. Select bake, set temperature 350 f, timer for 60 minutes. Press start to preheat the oven.
3. In a large mixing bowl, whisk eggs with pepper and salt. Add 1 cup cheese, bacon, and hash browns and mix well.
4. Pour egg mixture into the prepared casserole dish and sprinkle with remaining cheese.
5. Bake for 60 minutes or until the top is golden brown.
6. Slice and serve.

3.Mexican Breakfast Frittata

Prep time: 10 minutes

Cook time: 25 minutes

Yield: 6 servings

Ingredients:

- 8 eggs, scrambled
- 1/2 cup cheddar cheese, grated
- 3 scallions, chopped
- 1/3 lb. tomatoes, sliced
- 1 green pepper, chopped
- 1/2 cup salsa
- 2 tsp. taco seasoning
- 1 tbsp. olive oil
- 1/2 lb. ground beef
- Pepper
- Salt

Directions:

1. Spray a baking dish with cooking spray and set it aside.
2. Insert wire rack in rack position 6. Select bake, set temperature 375 f, timer for 25 minutes. Press start to preheat the oven.
3. Heat oil in a pan over medium heat. Add ground beef to a pan and cook until brown.
4. Add salsa, taco seasoning, scallions, and green pepper into the pan and stir well.
5. Transfer meat into the prepared baking dish. Arrange tomato slices on top of the meat mixture.

6. In a bowl, whisk eggs with cheese, pepper, and salt. Pour egg mixture over meat mixture and bake for 25 minutes.

7. Serve and enjoy.

4.Perfect Brunch Baked Eggs

Total time: 30 min

Prep time: 10 minutes

Cook time: 20 minutes

Servings: 4

Ingredients:

- 4 eggs
- 1/2 cup parmesan cheese, grated
- 2 cups marinara sauce
- Pepper
- Salt

Directions:

1. Spray with cooking spray on four shallow baking dishes and set aside.

2. Wire rack insertion at rack position 6. Pick bake, set temperature to 390 f, 20-minute timer. To preheat the oven, press start.

3. Divide the marinara sauce into four plates for baking.

4. Through each baking dish, split the egg. Sprinkle the eggs with cheese, pepper, and salt and bake for 20 minutes.

5. Enjoy and serve.

5. Green Chile Cheese Egg Casserole

Prep time: 10 minutes

Cook time: 40 minutes

Yield: 12 servings

Ingredients:

- 12 eggs
- 8 oz. can green chilies, diced
- 6 tbsp. butter, melted
- 3 cups cheddar cheese, shredded
- 2 cups curd cottage cheese
- 1 tsp. baking powder
- 1/2 cup flour
- Pepper
- Salt

Directions:

1. Spray a 9*13-inch baking dish with cooking spray and set aside.
2. Insert wire rack in rack position 6. Select bake, set temperature 350 f, timer for 40 minutes. Press start to preheat the oven.
3. In a large mixing bowl, beat eggs until fluffy. Add baking powder, flour, pepper, and salt.
4. Stir in green chilies, butter, cheddar cheese, and cottage cheese.
5. Pour egg mixture into the prepared baking dish and bake for 40 minutes.
6. Slice and serve.

6.Kale Zucchini Bake

Prep time: 10 minutes

Cook time: 30 minutes

Yield: 4 servings

Ingredients:

- 1 onion, chopped
- 1 cup zucchini, shredded and squeezed out all liquid
- 1/2 tsp. dill
- 1/2 tsp. oregano
- Six eggs
- 1 cup cheddar cheese, shredded
- 1 cup kale, chopped
- 1/2 tsp. basil
- 1/2 tsp. baking powder
- 1/2 cup almond flour
- 1/2 cup milk
- 1/4 tsp. salt

Directions:

1. With cooking oil, spray a 9*9-inch baking dish and put it aside.

2. Wire rack insertion at rack position 6. Pick bake, set temperature to 375 f, 35-minute timer. To preheat the oven, press start.

3. Whisk the eggs with the milk in a large mixing cup. Add the remaining ingredients, stirring until well mixed.

4. In the prepared baking dish, add in the egg mixture and bake for 35 minutes.

5. Slicing and cooking.

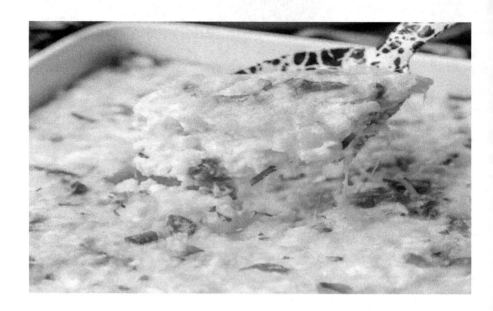

7.Cheesy Breakfast Casserole

Total time: 1 hour 10 min

Prep time: 10 min

Cook time: 60 min

Yield: 6 servings

Ingredients:

- 4 eggs
- 2 cups of milk
- 1 1/2 cup cheddar cheese, shredded
- Five bread slices, cut into cubes
- Pepper
- Salt

Directions:

1. Spray one 1/2-quart of baking dish and set aside with cooking spray.

2. Layer cubes of bread and alternately shredded cheese in a prepared baking dish.

3. Whisk the eggs with sugar, pepper and salt in a bowl and spill over the bread mixture. Put in the refrigerator overnight with a baking bowl.

4. Insert wire rack in place of rack 6. Pick bake, set temperature to 350 f, 60-minute timer. To preheat the oven, press start.

5. Take the baking dish out of the oven. For 60 minutes, roast.

6. Slicing and cooking.

8.Easy Hash Brown Breakfast Bake

Total time: 55 min

Prep time: 10 min

Cook time: 45 min

Yield: 8 servings

Ingredients:

- 8 eggs
- 1 cup cheddar cheese, shredded
- 1 lb. bacon slices, cooked and crumbled
- Pepper
- 30 oz. frozen cubed hash brown potatoes, thawed
- 2 cups of milk
- Salt

Directions:

1. Spray a 13*9-inch baking dish with cooking spray and set aside.
2. Insert wire rack in rack position 6. Select bake, set temperature 350 f, timer for 45 minutes. Press start to preheat the oven.
3. Add hash brown, bacon, and 1/2 cup cheese into the prepared baking dish.
4. In a bowl, whisk eggs with milk, pepper, and salt and pour over hash brown mixture. Sprinkle with remaining cheese and bake for 45 minutes.
5. Slice and serve.

9.Mexican Chiles Breakfast Bake

Total time: 50 min

Prep time: 10 min

Cook time: 40 min

Yield: 15 servings

Ingredients:

- Six eggs
- 20 oz. hash brown potatoes, shredded
- 1/4 tsp. ground cumin
- 1/2 cup milk
- 2 cups Mexican cheese, shredded
- 1 lb. pork sausage, cooked and crumbled
- 1 cup chunky salsa
- 28 oz. can whole green chilies
- Pepper
- Salt

Directions:

1. Spray a 13*9-inch baking dish with cooking spray and set aside.

2. Insert wire rack in rack position 6. Select bake, set temperature 350 f, timer for 40 minutes. Press start to preheat the oven.

3. Layer half potatoes, chilies, salsa, half sausage, and half cheese into the prepared baking dish. Cover with remaining sausage, potatoes, and cheese.

4. In a bowl, whisk eggs with milk, cumin, pepper, and salt and pour over potato mixture and bake for 40 minutes.

5. Serve and enjoy.

10.Delicious Amish Baked Oatmeal

Total time: 40 min

Prep time: 10 min

Cook time: 30 min

Yield: 8 servings

Ingredients:

- Two eggs
- 3 cups rolled oats
- 1 tsp. cinnamon
- 1 1/2 tsp. vanilla
- 1 1/2 tsp. baking powder
- 1/4 cup butter, melted
- 1/2 cup maple syrup
- 1 1/2 cups milk
- 1/4 tsp. salt

Directions:

1. Spray an 8*8-inch baking dish with cooking spray and set aside.
2. Insert wire rack in rack position 6. Select bake, set temperature 350 f, timer for 30 minutes. Press start to preheat the oven.
3. In a large bowl, whisk eggs with milk, cinnamon, vanilla, baking powder, butter, maple syrup, and salt. Add oats and mix well.
4. Pour mixture into the baking dish and bake for 30 minutes.
5. Slice and serve with warm milk and fruits.

11.Pork Sirloin Steak

Total time: 55 min

Prep time: 40 min

Cook time: 15 min

Yield: 2 servings

Ingredients:

- 1/2 onion
- 1 teaspoon ginger powder
- 1 teaspoon garlic powder
- 1 teaspoon ground cinnamon
- 1/2 teaspoon ground cardamom
- 1/2 - 1 teaspoon cayenne
- 1 teaspoon salt
- 1-pound boneless pork sirloin steaks

Directions:

1. Start by seasoning the steaks with pork loin. A generous amount of black pepper and salt, with a slight sprinkle of dried sage, is all you want to use. Don't be shy when it comes to seasoning. Before proceeding, making sure to season all sides of all the steaks properly.

2. On medium to high heat, melt a tablespoon of butter in a skillet. I want to wait until the cooking and bubbling of the butter begins. This means that the entire pan is heavy. This recipe for pork loin steak requires butter, not cooking spray or grease. Cooking steaks in butter adds so much flavor to them, and I notice that juicy steaks are created in this way.

3. It's time to add the steaks when the pan is heated, and the butter is melting and fried. You can cook 1 or 2 of them at a time. Just make sure you're not

overfilling your plate. Leave it to cook until faint signs of browning begin to surface on the underside, then turn and cook on the other side. This is 4-5 minutes of cooking time on either side.

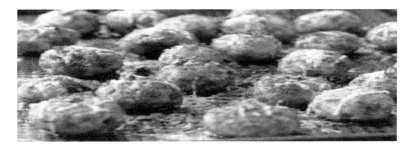

12.Chicken Meatballs with Cream Sauce and Cauliflower

Prep time: 40 min

Cook time: 15 min

Yield: 2 servings

Ingredients:

- 10 oz. Ground chicken
- 1 egg
- 2 oz. Grated parmesan cheese
- 1 teaspoon salt
- ½ teaspoon pepper
- 1 teaspoon dried basil
- 2 tablespoons sun-dried tomatoes in oil
- 1 tablespoon butter
- 1 lb. cauliflower
- 2 tablespoons butter for serving
- Cream sauce
- 1¼ cups coconut cream
- 1 tablespoon tomato paste
- 3 tablespoons finely chopped
- Fresh basil

Directions:

1. Combine the ground chicken ingredients and use a spoon to make 10 to 12 large balls (per pound). Following the manufacturer's instructions, ready the fryer. With a paper towel, gently coat the basket with elongated coconut oil and bake at 350 degrees for 10-13 minutes until lightly browned. Bring the oven back in and cook for another 4 to 5 minutes.

2. Place it on a plate after frying, then apply the cream and tomato paste. Let it cook over medium heat for 10 minutes.

3. With salt and pepper, season. Just before serving, add the fresh basil and cook the cauliflower for a few minutes in gently salted water. Serve alongside the chicken balls and cream sauce with a spoonful of sugar.

13. Shrimp Salad

Total time: 25 min

Prep time: 10 min

Cook time: 15 min

Yield: 2 servings

Ingredients:

- The salad
- 6 leaves lettuce
- 300 grams peeled shrimp
- 1 ½ tablespoon avocado oil
- ½ cup chopped celery
- 1 stalk chopped leek
- 4 tablespoons Greek yogurt

- 1 tablespoon coconut cream
- ½ teaspoon mint
- ½ teaspoon dried basil
- ¼ teaspoon chili powder
- 1 teaspoon lime juice

Directions:

1. Place the shrimp in the frying basket in one layer and air fried in the oven at 400 ° f for 10-14 minutes, depending on the size of the shrimp.

2. In a cup, mix together Greek yogurt, coconut milk, mint, dried basil, chili powder and lime juice.

3. Using the sliced celery and leek to place the fried shrimp in the dish. Combine the shrimp and vegetables before the dressing is covered.

4. Divide the lettuce and fill with the salad into separate portions.

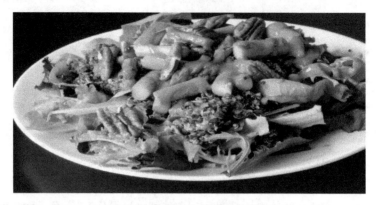

14.Maple Asparagus Salad with Pecans

Total time: 25 min

Prep time: 10 min

Cook time: 15 min

Yield: 4 servings

Ingredients:

- 10 medium asparagus spears
- ½ cup cherry tomatoes halved
- ½ cup chopped pecans
- ½ cup crumbled feta cheese
- 1-1/2 tablespoons coconut oil
- 1 tablespoon maple syrup

Directions:

1. Clean and cut the rough ends of the asparagus and spray coconut oil on the asparagus.

2. In an air fryer, place the asparagus in the oven. Cook at 360 degrees for 6 to 10 minutes to be crispy. In a cup, put the tomato halves, the diced pecans and the grated feta cheese.

3. In a shallow bowl, combine the coconut oil with the maple syrup and add the asparagus to the salad

mix. Pour over the salad with the dressing combination.

4. To ensure the ingredients are evenly covered, combine the lettuce.

15.Creamed Kale

Total time: 25 min

Prep time: 10 min

Cook time: 15 min

Yield: 4 servings

Ingredients:

- 1 10 ounces package frozen kale, thawed
- 1/2 cup onions, chopped
- 2 teaspoons garlic powder
- 4 ounces cream cheese, diced
- 1 teaspoon ground black pepper
- 1 teaspoon salt
- 1/2 teaspoon ground cinnamon
- 1/4 cup shredded goat cheese

Directions:

1. Grease a 6-inch pan and set it aside. Mix the kale, onion, garlic, diced cream cheese, salt, pepper and cinnamon in a medium bowl.

2. Pour into a greased pan and place the fryer at 350 ° f for 10 minutes. Open and mix the kale to mix the goat cheese through the kale and sprinkle the goat over it.

3. Set the fryer to 400 ° f for 5 minutes or until the cheese melts and turns brown.

16.Baked Zucchini

Total time: 25 min

Prep time: 10 min

Cook time: 15 min

Yield: 4 servings

Ingredients:

- 2 medium-large zucchinis
- 1 teaspoon coconut oil
- 2 teaspoons butter
- 1 teaspoon stevia
- 1/2 teaspoon nutmeg

Directions:

4. Rub the zucchinis with olive oil

5. Place the zucchinis in the air fryer. Cook for 40 minutes at 400 degrees.

6. Remove the zucchinis from the air fryer and allow them to cool.

7. Slice them open and load 1 teaspoon of butter and stevia and 1/4 teaspoon of nutmeg into each.

8. Cooking time may vary because every air fryer brand is different.

17.Roasted Broccoli Avocado Soup

Total time: 20 min

Prep time: 10 min

Cook time: 10 min

Yield: 4 servings

Ingredients:

- 1 head broccoli
- 1 tablespoon garlic powder

- 2 cups chicken stock or vegetable stock
- 1 avocado peeled and cubed
- 1/2 lemon juiced
- 1 tablespoon coconut oil
- Sea salt to taste
- Fresh ground pepper to taste

Directions:

9. Preheat the fryer to 390 degrees. Mix broccoli with garlic powder, salt and pepper and roast for 10 minutes. Carefully pour the broccoli with the other ingredients into the blender at high speed and puree until it is smooth.

10. Add salt and pepper as desired, add water too thin to desired consistency if necessary and heat slightly over medium heat. Serve immediately.

18.Herbed Tuna

Total time: 20 min

Prep time: 10 min

Cook time: 10 min

Yield: 2 servings

Ingredients:

- 8 oz. Sizzle fish tuna filets
- 1 teaspoon herbs
- 1/4 teaspoon sea salt
- 1/4 teaspoon black pepper
- 1/4 teaspoon smoked paprika
- 2 tablespoons coconut oil
- 1 tablespoon butter

Directions:

1. Using a paper towel to dry fillets and run the surface carefully to ensure there are no bones.
2. Spray the fish with coconut oil and brush it on the two sides of the solution.
3. On both sides of the fish, combine the seasoning and scatter.
4. Cook an air fryer for 5-8 minutes at 390 degrees. Starting with 5 minutes, I suggest testing the fish and adding another minute to the time before it quickly crumbles with a fork.
5. In the oven, heat the seasoned butter for 30 seconds and spill it over the fish before eating.

19. Sirloin Steak

Total time: 20 min

Prep time: 10 min

Cook time: 10 min

Yield: 2 servings

Ingredients:

- 2 sirloin steaks
- Two tablespoons steak seasoning
- Coconut oil

Directions:

1. Using a paper towel to dry fillets and run the surface carefully to ensure there are no bones.
2. Spray the fish with coconut oil and brush it on the two sides of the solution.
3. On both sides of the fish, combine the seasoning and scatter.
4. Cook an air fryer for 5-8 minutes at 390 degrees. Starting with 5 minutes, I suggest testing the fish and adding another minute to the time before it quickly crumbles with a fork.
5. In the oven, heat the seasoned butter for 30 seconds and spill it over the fish before eating.

20.Whole Chicken

Total time: 1 hour 5 min

Prep time: 05 min

Cook time: 60 min

Yield: 4 servings

Ingredients:

- 1 (4-pound) whole chicken,

- 1 tablespoon coconut oil
- ¼ tablespoon kosher salt
- ½ teaspoon freshly ground black pepper
- ½ teaspoon garlic powder
- ½ teaspoon paprika (I prefer smoked paprika)
- ¼ teaspoon dried mint
- ¼ teaspoon dried oregano
- ¼ teaspoon dried thyme

Directions:

1. Mix all of the spices into a paste with the oil and spread them all over the chicken.
2. Spray a basket of air fryers with an oil spray. Place the chicken in the basket face down and cook for 50 minutes at 360f.
3. Turn the chicken upside down and cook 10 minutes more.
4. Verify that there is an internal temperature of 165f in the breast chicken. Slice and serve.

21.Mini Sweet Pepper Poppers

Total time: 30 min

Prep time: 10 min

Cook time: 20 min

Yield: 4 (2 per servings)

Ingredients:

- 8 mini sweet peppers
- 4 ounces of full-Fat: cream cheese, softened
- 4 slices of sugar-free bacon, cooked and crumbled
- 1/4 cup of shredded pepper jack cheese

Directions:

1. Cut the pepper tops and slice on half lengthwise each. To cut seeds and membranes using a small knife.

2. Put together the cream cheese, bacon, and pepper jack in a shallow bowl.

3. In each sweet pepper, put 3 teaspoons of the mixture and press smoothly hard—place in basket fryer.

4. Set the temperature to 400° F, and set the timer for eight minutes.

5. Serve and enjoy!

22.Spicy Spinach Artichoke Dip

Total time: 30 min

Prep time: 10 min

Cook time: 20 min

Yield: (2 per servings)

Ingredients:

- 10 ounces of frozen spinach, drained and thawed
- 1 (14-ounce) can of artichoke hearts, drained and chopped
- 1/4 cup of chopped pickled jalapenos
- 8 ounces of full-Fat: cream cheese, softened
- 1/4 cup of full-Fat: mayonnaise
- 1/4 cup of full-Fat: sour cream
- 1/2 teaspoon of garlic powder
- ¼ cup of grated Parmesan cheese
- 1 cup of shredded pepper jack cheese

Directions:

1. In a 4-cup baking dish, combine the ingredients. In the Air Fryer, bring the basket in.

2. Fix the temperature for 10 minutes to 320° F and adjust the timer.

3. Start with an orange, then a bubble. Serve new and savor it!

23.Personal Mozzarella Pizza Crust

Total time: 30 min

Prep time: 10 min

Cook time: 20 min

Yield: (1per servings)

Ingredients:

- 1/2 cup of shredded whole-milk mozzarella cheese
- 2 tablespoons of blanched finely ground almond flour
- 1 tablespoon of full-Fat: cream cheese
- 1 large egg white

Directions:

1. In a medium microwave-safe bowl, place the mozzarella, almond flour, and cream cheese. Microwave that lasted 30 seconds. Stir until the dough ball forms smoothly. Add egg white and stir until the dough forms soft and round.

2. Press the crust of a 6 round pizza.

3. Cut a piece of parchment to fit your Air Fryer basket and place the crust on the parchment.

4. Set the temperature to 350° F and adjust the timer for 10 minutes.

5. Flip over the crust after 5 minutes and place any desired toppings at this time. Continue to cook until golden. Serve immediately.

24.Garlic Cheese Bread

Total time: 20 min

Prep time: 10 min

Cook time: 10 min

Yield: (2per servings)

Ingredients:

- 1 cup of shredded mozzarella cheese
- 1/4 cup of grated Parmesan cheese
- 1 large egg
- 1/2 teaspoon of garlic powder

Directions:

1. In a wide bowl, combine the ingredients. To suit your Air Fryer basket, cut a piece of parchment. Press the mixture in a circle onto the parchment, and put it in the Air Fryer basket.
2. Fix the temperature for 10 minutes to 350° F and adjust the timer.
3. Serve it warm and eat it!

25.Crustless Three-Meat Pizza

Total time: 20 min

Prep time: 10 min

Cook time: 10 min

Yield: (2per servings)

Ingredients:

- 1/2 cup of shredded mozzarella cheese

- 7 slices of pepperoni
- 1/4 cup of cooked ground sausage
- 2 slices of sugar-free bacon, cooked and crumbled
- 1 tablespoon of grated Parmesan cheese
- 2 tablespoons of low-carb, sugar-free pizza sauce for dipping

Directions:

1. Cover the bottom of the cake pan with mozzarella. Put the pepperoni, sausage, and bacon on top of the cheese and sprinkle with the Parmesan. Place the pan in the basket of the Air Fryer.

2. Change the temperature to 400° F and set a 5-minute timer.

3. Cut until the cheese is crispy and bubbling. Serve warm with a pizza sauce for dipping.

26.Smoky BBQ Roasted Almonds

Total time: 20 min

Prep time: 10 min

Cook time: 10 min

Yield: (2per servings)

Ingredients:

- 1 cup of raw almonds
- 2 teaspoons of coconut oil
- 1 teaspoon of chili powder
- 1/4 teaspoon of cumin
- 1/4 teaspoon of smoked paprika
- 1/4 teaspoon of onion powder

Directions:

1. Put all the ingredients in a big bowl before the almonds are filled equally with oil and spices. Put the almonds in the Air Fryer box.
2. Fix the temperature for 6 minutes to 320° F and adjust the timer.
3. Halfway through the cooking process, remove the basket from the fryer. Enable it to totally cool off.

27.Beef Jerky

Total time: 20 min

Prep time: 10 min

Cook time: 10 min

Yield: (2per servings)

Ingredients:

- 1-pound of flat iron beef, thinly sliced
- 1/4 cup of soy sauce
- 2 teaspoons of Worcestershire sauce
- 1/4 teaspoon of crushed red pepper flakes
- 1/4 teaspoon of garlic powder
- 1/4 teaspoon of onion powder

Directions:

1. Place all the ingredients in a plastic bag or sealed container and marinate for 2 hours in the fridge.
2. On the Air Fryer rack, placed each jerky slice into a single sheet.
3. Fix the temperature to 160° F and for 4 hours, set the timer.
4. Up to 1 week of storage in airtight containers.

28.Pork Rind Nachos

Total time: 20 min

Prep time: 10 min

Cook time: 10 min

Yield: (2per servings)

Ingredients:

- 1-ounce of pork rinds
- 4 ounces of shredded cooked chicken
- 1/2 cup of shredded Monterey jack cheese
- 1/4 cup of sliced pickled jalapeños
- 1/4 cup of guacamole
- 1/4 cup of full-Fat: sour cream

Directions:

In a 6' round baking tray, put pork rinds. Fill with grilled chicken and cheese jack from Monterey. Place the Air Fryer in the basket with the plate.

Set the temperature to 370 degrees F and set the timer before the cheese is melted or for 5 minutes.

With jalapeños, guacamole, and sour cream, enjoy right now.

29.Ranch Roasted Almonds

Total time: 20 min

Prep time: 10 min

Cook time: 10 min

Yield: (2per servings)

Ingredients:

- 2 cups of raw almonds
- 2 tablespoons of unsalted butter, melted
- 1/2 (1-ounce) ranch dressing mix packet

46

Directions:

1. To coat equally, stir the almonds in a large bowl of butter. Place almonds in the basket for Air Fryer Sprinkle ranch blend and sprinkle over almonds.

2. Fix the temperature for 6 minutes to 320° F and adjust the timer.

3. Shake the basket two or three times during training.

4. For at least 20 minutes, let it cool down. Almonds can become smooth during refrigeration to become crunchier. Place it in an air-tightened container for up to 3 days.

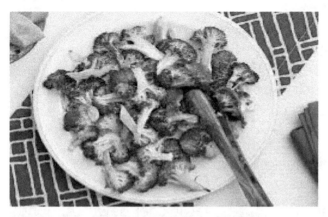

30.Loaded Roasted Broccoli

Total time: 20 min

Prep time: 10 min

Cook time: 10 min

Yield: (2per servings)

Ingredients:

- 3 cups of fresh broccoli florets
- 1 tablespoon of coconut oil
- 1/2 cup of shredded sharp Cheddar cheese
- 1/4 cup of full-Fat: sour cream
- 4slices of sugar-free bacon, cooked and crumbled
- 1 scallion, sliced

Directions:

1. Take the broccoli and drizzle it with coconut oil in the Air Fryer bowl.
2. Switch the temperature to 350 degrees F and set the timer for a further 10 minutes.
3. During exercise, toss a basket two or three times, or stop burning spots.

4. Remove from the fryer as the top begins to crisp the broccoli. Garnish with the melted cheese, sour cream, and crumbled bacon and scallion slices.

31.Scrumptious Leg of Lamb

Preparation time: 5 minutes

Cooking time: 1 hour

Servings: 4

Ingredients:

- 1 1/4 kg leg of lamb
- 1 tablespoon olive oil
- A pinch of sea salt
- Pepper

Directions:

1. Season the lamb's leg with salt and pepper and put it in the basket of the fryer.
2. Cook at 360 degrees for 20 minutes, turn the lamb's leg over and cook for a further 20 minutes.
3. Using roasted potatoes to serve.

32.Chinese Style Pork Chops

Preparation time: 15 minutes

Cooking time: 20 minutes

Servings: 4

Ingredients:

- 450g Pork chops
- ¾ cup corn/potato starch
- 1 egg white
- ¼ tsp. Freshly ground black pepper
- ½ tsp. Kosher salt

- For the stir fry:
- 2 green onions, sliced
- 2 jalapeno peppers, seeds removed and sliced
- 2 tbsp. Peanut oil
- ¼ tsp. Freshly ground pepper and kosher salt to taste

Directions:

1. Brush or spray with oil on the basket of your toast oven air fryer.

2. Next, mix the egg, salt and black pepper until it's frothy. Break up the pork chops and wipe the meat dry using a clean kitchen towel.

3. Toss the cutlets until evenly covered in the frothy egg mixture. For 30 minutes, cover and marinate.

4. Place the pork chops in a separate bowl and pour in the starch of corn/potato to ensure that each culet is dredged thoroughly. Shake off the extra corn/potato starch and place the prepared basket with the pork chops.

5. Set the air fryer toast oven to 360 degrees F and cook for 9 minutes, then shake the basket every 2-3 minutes, and if necessary, spray or brush the cutlets with more oil.

6. Increase the temperature to 400 degrees F and cook for another 6 minutes or until the chops are crisp.

7. Heat a wok or pan until incredibly hot over high heat. Apply all the ingredients for the stir fry and sauté for a minute.

8. Attach the pork chops you've fried and toss them with the stir fry.

9. Cook for another minute to guarantee that the stir-fry ingredients are uniformly mixed with the pork chops.

Enjoy!

33.Cinco De Mayo Pork Taquitos

Preparation time: 20 minutes

Cooking time: 15 minutes

Servings: 5

Ingredients:

- 400g cooked and shredded pork tenderloin
- 10 flour tortillas2 ½ cups mozzarella, shredded
- 1 lemon, juiced
- Sour cream
- Salsa
- Cooking spray

Directions:

1. Set your air fryer toast oven to 380 degrees f.
2. Squeeze the lemon juice over the shredded pork and mix well to combine.
3. Divide the tortillas into two and microwave, I batch at a time, covered with a slightly damp paper towel, so they don't become hard, for 15 seconds.
4. Divide the pork and cheese among the 10 tortillas.
5. Gently but tightly roll up all the tortillas.
6. Line your air fryer toast oven's pan with kitchen foil and arrange the tortillas on the pan.
7. Spray the tortillas with the cooking spray and cook for about 10 minutes, turning them over halfway through cook time.

8. Serve hot and enjoy!

34.Tangy Smoked Pork Chops with Raspberry Sauce

Preparation time: 15 minutes

Cooking time: 25 minutes

Servings: 4

Ingredients:

- 4 medium-sized smoked pork chops
- 1 cup panko bread crumbs
- 2 eggs
- ¼ cup all-purpose flour
- ¼ cup milk
- 1 cup pecans, finely chopped
- 1/3 cup aged balsamic vinegar
- 2 tbsp. Raspberry jam, seedless
- 1 tbsp. Orange juice concentrate
- 2 tbsp. Brown sugar

Directions:

1. Set your air fryer toast oven to 400 degrees f and spray/brush your air fryer toast oven's basket gently with oil.
2. Combine the milk and the eggs using a fork.
3. Mix the panko bread crumbs with the finely diced pecan in a separate bowl and place the flour in a third bowl.
4. Coat, one chop of pork at a time, of starch, brushing off the surplus.

5. Next, dunk the milk mixture and gently coat the crumb mixture on both sides. Gently pat to make the crumbs bind to the pork chops.

6. In the prepared basket, place the pork chops in one layer, spray lightly with cooking oil and cook for about 15 minutes, turning the chops halfway through the cooking time.

7. Combine all of the remaining ingredients in a pan over low-medium heat while the chops are frying. Carry to a boil until it thickens, then cook for 5-8 minutes.

8. Take out the chops and serve hot with the raspberry sauce.

9. Enjoy!

35. Air fryer toast oven bacon

Preparation time: 5 minutes

Cooking time: 15 minutes

Servings: 6

Ingredients:

- 1/2 package (16 ounces) bacon

Directions:

1. Preheat to 390° f with your air fryer toast cooker.

2. Arrange the bacon in the basket of the fryer in a single layer and cook for 8 minutes.

3. Flip the bacon over and cook for 7 more minutes or until crisp.

4. To drain excess grease, move it to a paper-lined tray.

5. Enjoy warm!

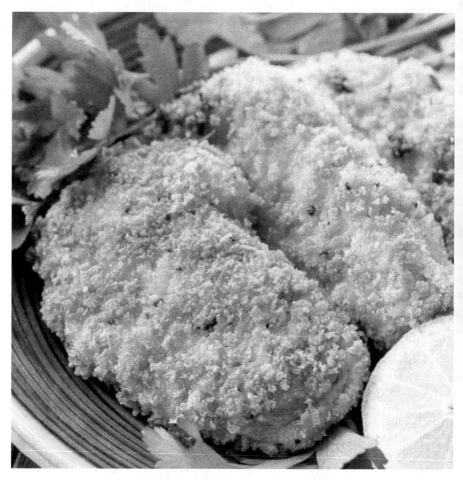

36.Italian Pork Milanese

Preparation time: 20 minutes

Cooking time: 10 minutes

Servings: 46

Ingredients:

- 6 pork chops, center-cut
- 2 eggs
- 2 tbsp. Water
- 1 cup panko bread crumbs seasoned with salt and black pepper

- ½ cup all-purpose flour
- 2 tbsp. Extra virgin olive oil
- Parmesan cheese, for serving (optional)
- For arugula salad:
- 1 bag fresh arugula
- 2 tbsp. Freshly squeezed lemon juice
- 1 tsp. Dijon mustard
- 1/8 cup extra virgin olive oil
- Freshly ground black pepper and sea salt to taste

Directions:

1. To pound each chop of pork into 1/4 inch cutlets, use a mallet or rolling pin.
2. Season well with salt and pepper, then dip the flour into each cutlet. Shake the waste off.
3. In a small cup, whisk the eggs with water and dip the floured cutlets in the mixture, then roll them into the bread crumbs.
4. For all of the chops, do this and put it aside.
5. Set 380 degrees f for your air fryer toast oven.
6. Brush the breaded pork chops gently with olive and place the toast oven basket in one sheet on your air fryer. Cook for 3-5 minutes or until golden and crisp, then flip the chops and cook for another 3-5 minutes.
7. Meanwhile, in a large bowl, cook the salad by mixing the mustard, lemon juice, salt and pepper. With the vinaigrette, toss the arugula until finely covered.
8. Serve the arugula salad and top with crisp cutlets and parmesan cheese (optional). Enjoy!

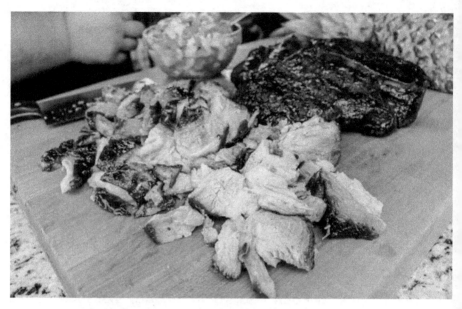

37.Jamaican Jerk Pork Roast

Preparation time: 10 minutes

Cooking time: 1 hour 10 minutes

Servings: 10

Ingredients:

- 1800g pork shoulder
- 1 tbsp. Olive oil
- 1/4 cup Jamaican jerk spice blend
- 1/2 cup beef broth

Directions:

1. Set your air fryer to 400 degrees f and brown roast on both sides for 4 minutes on each side after rubbing the oil and seasoning.

2. Then decrease the temperature to 350 degrees f and bake for 1 hour, then remove from the fryer.

3.

4. Shred and serve.

38.Tasty and Moist Air Fryer Toast Oven Meatloaf

Preparation time: 20 minutes

Cooking time: 20 minutes

Servings: 4

Ingredients:

- 450 g lean minced meat
- 250 ml tomato sauce
- 1 small onion, finely chopped
- 1 tsp. Minced garlic
- 5 tbsp. Ketchup
- 1 tbsp. Worcestershire sauce
- 1/3 cup cornflakes crumbs
- 3 tsp. Brown sugar
- 1 ½ tsp. Freshly ground black pepper
- 1 ½ tsp. Sea salt
- 1 tsp. Dried basil
- ½ tsp. Freshly chopped parsley

Directions:

1. Combine the minced beef, corn flakes, chopped onion, garlic, basil, salt, pepper, and 3/4 of the tomato sauce in a large bowl. To blend and ensure that all the ingredients are mixed equally, use your hands.

2. Take your two shallow loaf pans and brush them loosely with vegetable oil. Divide the mixture of the meatloaf into two loaf pans.

3. Set the oven to 360 degrees f for your air fryer breakfast.

4. Combine the remainder of the tomato sauce, ketchup, Worcestershire sauce and brown sugar in a cup for the glaze. On the top and sides of the two loaves, rub this glaze blend.

5. Place the loaf pans, too, in the fryer. Cook and re-apply the glaze on the top and sides of the meatloaves for 10 minutes.

6. Cook for a further 10 minutes, twice in between, adding the glaze.

7. Sprinkle with the new parsley and cut the two loaf pans.

8. Before extracting the loaves from the loaf pans, let them stand for 3 minutes.

9. With mashed potatoes and a green salad, serve the perfectly moist and delicious meatloaf.

10. Enjoy!

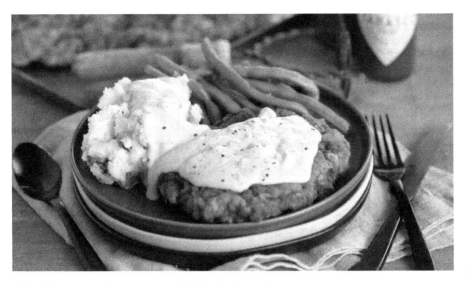

39.Classic Country Fried Steak

Preparation time: 15 minutes

Cooking time: 20 minutes

Servings: 2

Ingredients:

- 2 x 200g sirloin steaks
- 1 cup panko bread crumbs seasoned with kosher salt and freshly ground pepper
- 1 cup all-purpose flour
- 3 eggs, lightly beaten
- 1 tsp. Garlic powder
- 1 tsp. Onion powder
- For the sausage gravy:
- 150g ground sausage meat
- 2 cups milk
- 2 ½ tbsp. Flour
- 1 tsp. Freshly ground black pepper

Directions:

11. To pound the two steaks up to 1/2 - 1/4 inches thick, use a mallet or rolling pin.

12. In three separate shallow containers, placed the flour, egg and panko.

13. Dredge the steak in the flour first, then the egg and finally the bread crumbs then set them aside on a pan.

14. Brush the basket gently with oil from your air fryer toast oven, and then put the two breaded steaks on the basket.

15. Set the oven to 370 degrees f for the air fryer toast and cook the steak for 12 minutes, flipping once halfway through the cooking time.

16. Meanwhile, prepare the gravy by frying the sausage meat over medium-low heat in a pan until it browns uniformly. Drain the extra fat and reserve it in the pan for around a tablespoon or two.

17. Stir in the flour until well mixed, then, little by little, pour in the milk, stirring all the while.

18. For 3 minutes, season with freshly ground pepper and boil until the gravy is good and thick.

19. Using the sauce and some fluffy mashed potatoes to eat the steak. Yum!

40. Bourbon Infused Bacon Burger

Preparation time: 45 minutes

Cooking time: 30 minutes

Servings: 2

Ingredients:

- 300g 80:20 lean ground beef
- 3 strips maple bacon, halved

- 1 small onion, minced
- 1 tbsp. Bourbon
- 2 tbsp. Bbq sauce
- 2 tbsp. Brown sugar
- 2 slices Monterey jack cheese
- Freshly ground black pepper, to taste
- Salt, to taste
- 2 burger rolls
- Sliced tomato for serving
- Torn lettuce, for serving
- For the sauce:
- 2 tbsp. Mayonnaise
- 2 tbsp. Bbq sauce
- ¼ tsp. Sweet paprika
- Freshly ground black pepper, to taste

Directions:

1. Set your air fryer toast oven to 390 degrees F and pour around 1/2 cup of water into your air fryer toast oven's bottom drawer. This causes the smoking/burning grease to trickle away.

2. Mix the bourbon with the sugar. Arrange the strips of bacon in the basket of your air fryer toast oven and spray the tops with the sugar-bourbon mixture. Cook for 4 minutes, change the strips and brush with more sugar-bourbon mix and cook until brown and super crisp for 4 more minutes.

3. Meanwhile, the ground beef, chopped onion, salt, pepper and bbq sauce are mixed to create the burgers. To mix well, use your hands to make 2 burger patties.

4. If you like your burgers well cooked, set the air fryer toast oven at 370 degrees f and cook the burgers for 20 minutes, or 12-15 minutes if you like them medium-rare. Halfway into cooking time, flip the burgers.

5. Meanwhile, mix all the sauce ingredients in a bowl and stick them in the fridge to produce the sauce.

6. Cover each burger with a slice of Monterey Jack cheese for one minute of your cooking time. To keep the cheese from being blown away in the fryer, bind the cheese to the patty using a toothpick.

7. Cut each roll and spread the sauce on the sliced halves of the rolls to assemble the burger. Place one half of the burger and cover it with the bacon, tomatoes, lettuce and the other half of the roll. Enjoy!

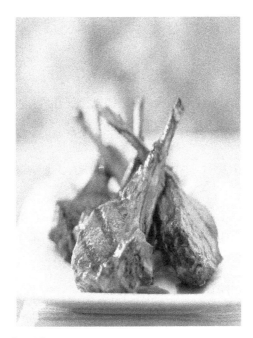

41.Glazed Lamb Chops

Preparation time: 10 minutes

Cooking time: 15 minutes

Servings: 4

Ingredients:

- 1 tablespoon dijon mustard
- ½ tablespoon fresh lime juice
- 1 teaspoon honey
- ½ teaspoon olive oil
- Salt and ground black pepper, as required
- 4 (4-ounce) lamb loin chops

Directions:

1. In a black pepper large bowl, mix the mustard, lemon juice, oil, honey, salt, and black pepper.

2. Add the chops and coat with the mixture generously.

3. Place the chops onto the greased "sheet pan."

4. Press the "power button" of the ninja food digital air fry oven and turn the dial to select the "air bake" mode.

5. Press the time button and again turn the dial to set the cooking time to 15 minutes.

6. Now push the temp button and rotate the dial to set the temperature at 390 degrees f.

7. Press the "start/pause" button to start.

8. When the unit beeps to show that it is preheated, open the lid.

9. Insert the "sheet pan" in the oven.

10. Flip the chops once halfway through.

11. Serve hot.

42. Buttered Leg of Lamb

Preparation time: 15 minutes

Cooking time: 1¼ hours

Servings: 8

Ingredients:

- 1 (2¼-pound) boneless leg of lamb
- 3 tablespoons butter, melted
- Salt and ground black pepper, as required
- 4 fresh rosemary sprigs

Directions:

1. Rub with butter on the leg of the lamb and sprinkle with salt and black pepper.

2. Wrap a leg of lamb with sprigs of rosemary.

3. "Press the ninja foodie digital air fry oven's "power button" and turn the dial to select the mode for "air fry.

4. To set the cooking time to 75 minutes, press the time button and change the dial once again.

5. Now press the temp button to set the temperature at 300 degrees f and rotate the dial.

6. To start, press the 'start/pause' button.

7. "Open the "air fry basket" lid and grease when the machine beeps to indicate that it is preheated.

8. Arrange the leg of lamb into an "air fry basket" and insert it in the oven.

9. Remove from the oven and put the lamb's leg on a cutting board before slicing for about 10 minutes.

10. Split into bits of the appropriate size and serve.

43.Glazed Lamb Meatballs

Preparation time: 20 minutes

Cooking time: 30 minutes

Servings: 8

Ingredients:

- For meatballs:
- ½ cup Ritz crackers, crushed
- Salt and ground black pepper, as required
- 1 (5-ounce) can evaporate milk
- 2 large eggs, beaten lightly
- 1 tablespoon dried onion, minced
- 1 teaspoon maple syrup

- 2 pounds lean ground lamb
- 2/3 cup quick-cooking oats
- For sauce:
- 1/3 cup sugar
- 1/3 cup orange marmalade
- 1-2 tablespoons sriracha
- 1/3 cup maple syrup
- 1 tablespoon Worcestershire sauce
- 2 tablespoons cornstarch
- 2 tablespoons soy sauce

Directions:

1. For meatballs: Put all the ingredients in a large bowl and mix until well mixed.
2. From the mixture, produce 11/2-inch balls.
3. Add half of the meatballs in a single layer to the greased "sheet pan."
4. "Press the ninja foodie digital air fry oven's "power button" and turn the dial to select the mode for "air fry.
5. To set the cooking time to 15 minutes, click the time button and change the dial once again.
6. Now press the temp button to set the temperature at 380 degrees f and rotate the dial.
7. To start, press the 'start/pause' button.
8. Open the lid when the device beeps to demonstrate that it is preheated.
9. Place the' sheet pan' in the oven.
10. Halfway through, turn the meatballs once.

11. Remove the meatballs from the oven and transfer them to a dish.

12. Repeat with the meatballs that remain.

13. Meanwhile, for sauce, put all the ingredients in a small pan: over medium heat and cook until thickened, stirring constantly.

14. Serve the meatballs with sauce on top.

44.Oregano Lamb Chops

Preparation time: 10 minutes

Cooking time: 30 minutes

Servings: 4

Ingredients:

- 4 lamb chops
- 1 garlic clove, peeled
- 1 tbsp. plus
- 2 tsp. olive oil
- ½ tbsp. oregano
- ½ tbsp. thyme
- Salt and black pepper to taste

Directions:

1. Preheat the fryer to 390 f for air. Coat the clove of garlic with 1 tsp. Place the olive oil in the air fryer for 10 minutes. Meanwhile, with the remaining olive oil, combine the herbs and seasonings.

2. Squeeze the hot roasted garlic clove into the herb mixture using a towel or a mitten, and stir to blend. Cover the lamb chops well with the mixture and put them in the oven for frying. For 8 to 12 minutes, cook. Serve it warm.

45.Lamb Steaks with Fresh Mint and Potatoes

Preparation time: 10 minutes

Cooking time: 25 minutes

Servings: 2

Ingredients:

- 2 lamb steaks
- 2 tbsp. Olive oil
- 2 garlic cloves, crushed
- Salt and pepper, to taste
- A handful of fresh thyme, chopped
- 4 red potatoes, cubed

Directions:

1. Using oil, garlic, salt, and black pepper to rub the steaks. In the fryer, put the thyme and place the steaks on top. Oil the chunks of the potato and sprinkle them with salt and pepper. Arrange the potatoes next to the steaks and cook for 14 minutes at 360 f, turning once halfway through the cooking process.

46.Lamb Kofta

Preparation time: 6 minutes

Cooking time: 12 minutes

Servings: 4

Ingredients:

- 1 pound ground lamb
- 1 tsp. cumin
- 2 tbsp. mint, chopped
- 1 tsp. garlic powder

- 1 tsp. onion powder
- 1 tbsp. ras el hanout
- ½ tsp. ground coriander
- 4 bamboo skewers
- Salt and black pepper to taste

Directions:

2. Lamb, cumin, garlic powder, mint, onion powder, ras el hanout, cilantro, salt and pepper are combined in a cup. Place on skewers and mold into sausage shapes. Marinate it in the fridge for 15 minutes.

3. Preheat to 380 f with your air fryer. Spray a basket of air fryers with cooking spray. Arrange the skewers in the basket of an air fryer. Cook for 8 minutes, turning once halfway through. Serve with dip with yogurt.

47.Crunchy Cashew Lamb Rack

Preparation time: 10 minutes

Cooking time: 30 minutes

Servings: 4

Ingredients:

- 3 oz. chopped cashews
- 1 tbsp. chopped rosemary
- 1 ½ lb. rack of lamb
- 1 garlic clove, minced
- 1 tbsp. breadcrumbs
- 1 egg, beaten
- 1 tbsp. olive oil
- Salt and pepper to taste

Directions:

1. Heat the air-freezer to 210 f. Combine the garlic with the olive oil and spray this mixture over the lamb. In a dish, blend the rosemary, cashews, and crumbs. Brush the lambs with the egg, then cover them with the cashew mixture. Place the lamb in the basket of an air fryer and cook for 25 minutes. Increase the heat to 390 f, and cook for an additional 5 minutes. Cover with foil and leave to rest before serving for a few minutes.

48.Oregano & Thyme Lamb Chops

Preparation time: 10 minutes

Cooking time: 30 minutes

Servings: 4

Ingredients:

- 4 lamb chops
- 1 garlic clove, peeled
- 1 tbsp. plus
- 2 tsp. olive oil
- ½ tbsp. oregano
- ½ tbsp. thyme
- ½ tsp. salt
- ¼ tsp. black pepper

Directions:

2. Preheat the fryer to 390 f for air. Coat the clove of garlic with 1 tsp. Olive oil and put for 10 minutes in the air fryer. With the remaining olive oil, combine the herbs and seasonings.

3. Squeeze the hot roasted garlic clove into the herb mixture using a towel or a mitten, and stir to blend.

Thoroughly coat the lamb chops with the mixture, and put in the air fryer. 12 minutes to cook.

49.Lamb Meatballs

Preparation time: 10 minutes

Cooking time: 40 minutes

Servings: 12

Ingredients:

- 1 ½ lb ground lamb
- ½ cup minced onion
- 2 tbsp. chopped mint leaves
- 3 garlic cloves, minced
- 2 tsp. paprika
- 2 tsp. coriander seeds
- ½ tsp. cayenne pepper
- 1 tsp. salt
- 1 tbsp. chopped parsley
- 2 tsp. cumin
- ½ tsp. ground ginger

Directions:

20. Soak 24 skewers in water until ready to use. Preheat the air fryer to 330 f. Combine all ingredients in a large bowl. Mix well with your hands until the herbs and spices are evenly distributed, and the mixture is well combined. Shape the lamb mixture into 12 sausage shapes around 2 skewers. Cook for 12 to 15 minutes, or until it reaches the preferred doneness. Served with tzatziki sauce and enjoy.

50.Thyme Lamb Chops with Asparagus

Preparation time: 10 minutes

Cooking time: 20 minutes

Servings: 4

Ingredients:

- 1 pound lamb chops
- 2tspolive oil
- 1½ tsp. chopped fresh thyme
- 1 garlic clove, minced
- Salt and black pepper to taste
- 4 asparagus spears, trimmed

Directions:

1. Preheat to 400 f with your air fryer. Spray a basket of air fryers with cooking spray.
2. Drizzle some olive oil with the asparagus, sprinkle with salt, and set aside with salt and black pepper, season the lamb. Brush and move the remaining olive oil to the cooking basket. Slide the basket out, transform the chops and add the asparagus. Cook for 10 minutes. For another 5 minutes, cook. Serve with thyme sprinkles.

51.Cornflakes French toast

Total time: 20 min

Prep time: 10 min

Cook time: 10 min

Yield: 2 servings

Ingredients:

- Bread slices (brown or white)
- 1 egg white for every 2 slices
- 1 tsp. of sugar for every 2 slices

- Crushed cornflakes

Directions:

1. Place two slices together, then trim them along the diagonal. In a bowl, whisk together the egg whites, then add a little sugar.

2. Immerse the bread triangles in this mixture and coat them with the crushed corn blossoms.

3. Preheat the Air Fryer at 180o C for 4 minutes. Place the triangles of coated bread in and close the box for frying. Let them cook for at least a further 20 minutes at the same temperature.

4. To get an even chef, turn the triangles over. Serve the slices of chocolate syrup.

52.Mint Galette

Total time: 10 min

Prep time: 5 min

Cook time: 5 min

Yield: 2 servings

Ingredients:

- 2 cups of mint leaves (Sliced fine)
- 2 medium potatoes boiled and mashed
- 1 ½ cup of coarsely crushed peanuts
- 3 tsp. of ginger finely chopped
- 1-2 tbsp. of fresh coriander leaves
- 2 or 3 green chilies finely chopped
- 1 ½ tbsp. of lemon juice
- Salt and pepper to the taste

Directions:

1. Mix the sliced mint leaves with the remaining ingredients in a clean dish. Shape this mixture into galettes that are flat and round.

2. Wet the galettes softly with sweat. Cover each peanut with each smashed galette.

3. Preheat the Air Fryer, at 160° Fahrenheit, for 5 minutes. Place the galettes in the frying bowl and let them steam at about the same temperature for another 25 minutes.

4. In order to get a cook that is even, keep turning them over. Using chutney, basil, or ketchup to serve.

53.Cottage Cheese Sticks

Total time: 10 min

Prep time: 5 min

Cook time: 5 min

Yield: 2 servings

Ingredients:

- 2 cups of cottage cheese
- 1 big lemon-juiced
- 1 tbsp. of ginger-garlic paste

For seasoning, use salt and red chili powder in small amounts

- ½ tsp. of carom
- One or two papadums
- 4 or 5 tbsp. of cornflour
- 1 cup of water

Directions:

1. Take the cheese and cut it into pieces that are long. Currently, a combination of lemon juice, red chili powder, spices, ginger garlic paste, and caramel is used as a marinade.

2. Marinate the slices of cottage cheese in the mixture for a bit, then wrap them in dry cornflour for about 20 minutes to set aside.

3. Take the papadum and cook it in a saucepan. Crush them until they are cooked into very tiny pieces. Take another bottle now and pour about 100 ml of water in it.

4. Loosen 2 tablespoons of cornflour in the water. Dip the cottage cheese pieces in this cornflour solution and roll them on to the bits of crushed papadum so that the papadum attaches to the cottage cheese.

5. Preheat the Air Fryer for 10 minutes at about 290 Fahrenheit. Then open the basket for the fryer and put the cottage cheese bits inside it. Cover the bowl well. Enable the fryer to sit at 160 ° for another 20 minutes.

6. Open the basket halfway through, and put a little of the cottage cheese around to allow for standard cooking. Until they're cooked, you can eat them with either ketchup or mint chutney. Serve and chutney with mint.

54.Palak Galette

Total time: 20 min

Prep time: 10 min

Cook time: 10 min

Yield: 2 servings

Ingredients:

- 2 tbsp. of garam masala

- 2 cups of Palak leaves
- 1 ½ cup of coarsely crushed peanuts
- 3 tsp. of ginger finely chopped
- 1-2 tbsp. of fresh coriander leaves
- 2 or 3 green chilies finely chopped
- 1 ½ tbsp. of lemon juice
- Salt and pepper to the taste

Directions:

1. Blend into a clean container with the ingredients. Shape this mixture into galettes that are smooth and round. Wet the galettes softly with sweat. Coat up each galette with smashed peanuts.

2. Preheat the Air Fryer, at 160° Fahrenheit, for 5 minutes. Place the galettes in the basket and let them cook for another 25 minutes at the same temperature. Go turn them over to cook them. Using ketchup or mint chutney to serve.

55.Spinach Pie

Total time: 10 min

Prep time: 5 min

Cook time: 5 min

Yield: 2 servings

Ingredients:

- 7 ounces of flour
- 2 tablespoons of butter
- 7ounces of spinach
- 1 tablespoon of olive oil
- 2 eggs

- 2 tablespoons of milk
- 3 ounces of cottage cheese
- Salt and black pepper to the taste
- 1 yellow onion, chopped

Directions:

1. In your food processor, mix flour and butter, 1 egg, milk, salt and pepper, combine properly, switch to a cup, knead, cover, and leave for 10 minutes.
2. Heat the pan with the oil over medium heat, add the spinach and onion, stir and simmer for 2 minutes.
3. Attach salt, pepper, cottage cheese, and leftover egg, stir well and heat up.
4. Divide the dough into 4 pieces, roll each piece, place it on a ramekin's rim, add the spinach filling over the dough, place the ramekins in your Air Fryer's basket, and cook at 360° F for 15 minutes.
5. Serve it sweet.

56.Balsamic Artichokes

Total time: 10 min

Prep time: 5 min

Cook time: 5 min

Yield: 7 servings

Ingredients:

- 4 big artichokes, trimmed
- Salt and black pepper to the taste
- 2 tablespoons of lemon juice
- ¼ cup of extra virgin olive oil
- 2 teaspoons of balsamic vinegar

- 1 teaspoon of oregano, dried
- 2 garlic cloves, minced

Directions:

1. Season the salt and pepper with the artichokes, rub them with half the oil and half the lemon juice, put them in your Air Fryer and cook at 360 ° F for 7 minutes.

2. Meanwhile, in a cup, combine the remaining lemon juice, vinegar, remaining oil, salt, pepper, garlic, and oregano and mix well.

3. Arrange the artichokes on a tray, coat them with a balsamic vinaigrette, and eat.

57.Cheesy Artichokes

Total time: 15 min

Prep time: 5 min

Cook time: 5 min

Yield: 7 servings

Ingredients:

- 14 ounces of canned artichoke hearts
- 8 ounces of cream cheese
- 16 ounces of parmesan cheese, grated
- 10 ounces of spinach
- ½ cup of chicken stock
- 8 ounces of mozzarella, shredded
- ½ cup of sour cream
- 3 garlic cloves, minced
- ½ cup of mayonnaise
- 1 teaspoon of onion powder

Directions:

1. In a saucepan appropriate for your Air Fryer, blend artichokes with stock, garlic, spinach, cream cheese, sour cream, onion powder and mayo, put in the Air Fryer, and cook for 6 minutes at 350 °F.

2. Apply the mozzarella and parmesan and then stir well and eat.

58.Artichokes and Special Sauce

Total time: 15 min

Prep time: 5 min

Cook time: 5 min

Yield: 2 servings

Ingredients:

- 2 artichokes, trimmed
- A drizzle of olive oil
- 2 garlic cloves, minced
- 1 tablespoon of lemon juice

For the sauce:

- ¼ cup of coconut oil
- ¼ cup of extra virgin olive oil
- 3 anchovy fillets
- 3 garlic cloves

Directions:

1. Mix the artichokes with the oil, 2 cloves of garlic and lemon juice in a cup, toss well, move to your Air Fryer, and cook for 6 minutes at 350 ° F and split between plates.

2. Mix coconut oil with anchovy, 3 garlic cloves, and olive oil in your food processor, blend very well, drizzle with artichokes and eat.

59.Beet Salad and Parsley Dressing

Total time: 25 min

Prep time: 10 min

Cook time: 25 min

Yield: 4 servings

Ingredients:

- 4 beets
- 2 tablespoons of balsamic vinegar
- A bunch of parsley, chopped
- Salt and black pepper to the taste
- 1 tablespoon of extra-virgin olive oil
- 1 garlic clove, chopped
- 2 tablespoons of capers

Directions:

1. Place the beets and cook at 360 ° F for 14 minutes in your Air Fryer.
2. Meanwhile, in a dish, mix the parsley, garlic, salt, pepper, olive oil, and capers, and whisk very well.
3. Move the beets to a cutting board, cool them down, slice them, and place them in a salad bowl.
4. All over the parsley dressing, apply vinegar and drizzle and eat.

60.Beets and Blue Cheese Salad

Total time: 25 min

Prep time: 10 min

Cook time: 25 min

Yield: 6 servings

Ingredients:

- 6 beets, peeled and quartered
- Salt and black pepper to the taste
- ¼ cup of blue cheese, crumbled
- 1 tablespoon of olive oil

Directions:

1. In the Air Fryer, place the beets, cook them at 350 ° F for 14 minutes and then move them to a dish.

2. Apply the blue cheese, salt, pepper, and oil to the mixture, and then toss and eat.

61.Shrimp Pancakes

Preparation Time: 5 Minutes

Cooking Time: 15 Minutes

Servings: 10-12

Ingredients:

- 1 cup all-purpose flour
- 1 glass of water
- 3 beaten eggs
- 1 tablet chicken broth

Directions:

1. Boil the water and dissolve the chicken broth, let it cool and place the beaten eggs and the wheat flour, stir well until everything dissolves and a smooth mass fry the tablespoons and a little oil in the Tefal pan and keep the part in a baking dish.

2. Make the prawns taste and leave with a little sauce.

3. Top with pancakes and shrimp sauce and sprinkle with grated cheese. Do this until the last layers of grated cheese are ready.

4. Bake in the air fryer at 3600F for 15 minutes. Serve with white rice and salad.

62.Shrimps with Palmito

Preparation Time: 10 Minutes

Cooking Time: 30 Minutes

Servings: 4-8

Ingredients:

White Sauce:

- 1 cup grated Parmesan cheese
- 1 tbsp. butter
- 4 ½ lb shrimp
- ½ cup of olive oil
- Very minced garlic Striped onion
- 1 can of sour cream
- 1 can of sliced palm heart Grated Parmesan

Sauce:

- 1 onion, sliced
- Margarine and butter
- 2 cups milk
- 2 tbsp. of flour
- Salt to taste
- cheese for sprinkling

Preparation of the white sauce:

1. With the margarine and butter, lightly brown the onion.

2. In a blender, place the milk and wheat flour.

3. Add the onion which has been stewed.

4. Beat it all really well.

5. Bring this mixture to the fire and cook until a dense cream appears. Add the Parmesan cheese and butter and extract the white sauce from the heat. Reserve. Reserve.

6. Sauté the snails with garlic and onion in olive oil.

7. To the white sauce, add the sautéed shrimp and eventually add the palm kernel and milk, mixing it all very well.

8. Sprinkle plenty of Parmesan cheese on top, set in a greased refractory form. 9. Bake for 1520 minutes in the air-fryer at 3600F.

63.Gratinated Pawns with Cheese
Preparation Time: 10 Minutes

Cooking Time: 20 Minutes

Servings: 4

Ingredients:

- 2 ¼ lbs. clean, chopped prawns
- 1 tbsp. of fondor
- 1 tbsp. of oil
- 1 tbsp. butter
- 1 grated onion
- 5 tomatoes, beaten in a blender
- 1 tablet of crumbled shrimp broth
- 1 glass of light cream cheese
- 1 tbsp. of breadcrumbs
- 1 tbsp. Parmesan cheese

Directions:

1. Use one such fondor to season the prawns and reserve for 1 hour.

2. In the oil and butter combination, cook them.

3. Position them and set them aside in a refractory container.

4. Brown, the onion in the fat of the shrimp, add the tomatoes, a tablet of the shrimp broth and a cup of boiling water.

5. Bring to a boil, until just a touch, in a covered skillet.

6. Add the curd, then stir until it freezes.

7. Pour over the prawns and sprinkle the mixed breadcrumbs with the grated rib.

8. Parmesan cheese and placed it in a 400oF air fryer for 20 minutes or until golden brown.

64.Air fryer Crab

Preparation Time: 5 Minutes

Cooking Time: 10 Minutes

Servings: 20

Ingredients:

- 1 pound of crab meat 20 crab cones
- 2 onions
- 2 tomatoes
- 3 garlic cloves
- 1 bell pepper
- ½ glass of white vinegar
- 1 head of black pepper
- 1 head of cumin

- 1 small salt
- Olive oil to taste

Directions:

1. Place the onion that has been sliced until golden. Then, with 1/2 glass of vinegar, add the remaining spices (pepper, cumin, minced garlic).

2. Put in the green smell, the crushed tomatoes, and the cut pepper. Add the olive oil to taste when the seasoning is well done (at least 3 tablespoons).

3. Then add the meat to the crab and cook for 5 minutes.

4. Fill the crab cones, drizzle with grated Parmesan cheese and bake for 5 minutes in an air fryer at 3200 to melt the cheese.

65.Crab Balls

Preparation Time: 10 Minutes

Cooking Time: 20 Minutes

Servings: 2-4

Ingredients:

- 1 lb of crab Salt to taste Olive oil
- 2 cloves garlic, minced
- 1 chopped onion
- 3 tbsp. of wheat flour
- 1 tbsp. of parsley
- 1 fish seasoning
- 2 lemons
- 1 cup milk

Tarnish:

1. Wash the crab in the juice of 1 lemon.

2. Season with the juice of the other lemon, along with the salt and the prepared fish seasoning.

3. In a frying pan, sauté the onion and garlic with the sweet oil.

4. Mix the crab meat with the stir fry. 5. Let cook in this mixture for another 5 minutes.

6. Add the parsley.

7. Dissolve the flour in the milk and add it to the crab.

8. Stir constantly, until this mixture begins to come out of the pan.

9. Let cool, shape the meatballs, go through the beaten egg and breadcrumbs.

10. 1 beaten egg Bread crumbs Oil for frying

11. Fry in the air fryer at 4000F for 25 minutes.

66.Crab Empanada
Preparation Time: 15 Minutes

Cooking Time: 30 Minutes

Servings: 4-8

Ingredients:

- 1 small onion
- 1 tomato
- 1 small green pepper
- 1 lb of crab meat Seasoning ready for fish
- 1 tbsp. of oil Pastry dough

Directions:

1. In oil, sauté the chopped onion, tomato, and pepper.

2. Add the sauce and crab meat.

3. Cook, without stirring, until very dry so that it does not stick to the bottom of the pan.

4. Fill the cakes with the crab meat that has been prepared.

5. Fry it in an air fryer for 25 minutes at 4000F.

67.Crab Meat on Cabbage

Preparation Time: 10 Minutes

Cooking Time: 15 Minutes

Servings: 2-4

Ingredients:

- 1 pound shredded crab meat
- 1 pound cooked and minced dogfish
- 2 cups of cooked rice
- 1 small green cabbage
- Parsley and coriander
- Chile
- 2 tbsp. of palm oil

Directions:

1. In a little water, season and cook the dogfish.

2. Crush the broth that has been created when it is smooth and drink it. Add the crab meat, which should have been thawed already. Add the tomato sauce, palm oil, pepper and cooked rice.

3. In warm water, dissolve the starch and pour it into the mixture. Sharpen the mixture, taste the salt and brush on top with the chopped parsley and coriander.

4. Cook 6 whole leaves of cabbage separately, until al dente, in salted water.

5. Place the open leaves and crab cream with 2 tbsp. of cornstarch in a baking dish. Tomato sauce Bread crumbs Garlic fish inside.

7. Sprinkle with breadcrumbs and bake for 5 minutes in an air fryer at 3200F to brown.

68.Gratinated Cod
Preparation Time: 15 Minutes

Cooking Time: 45 Minutes

Servings: 4-8

Ingredients:

- 2 ¼ lb cod
- 1 red bell pepper
- 1 green bell pepper
- 1 onion
- 3 ripe tomatoes
- 2 cloves of garlic
- 1 cup black olives
- Oregano to taste

Cream:

- 1 cup catupiry cheese
- 1 can of cream
- ½ cup coconut milk

Mashed potatoes:

1. First, prepare the mashed potatoes, squeeze the potatoes and, with the potatoes still very sweet, add the butter and cream, mix well and add salt to taste.

2. On a high ovenproof plate, put this puree. Then arrange yourself like a pie crust. Make the stir fry with

the already desalted cod (soak the day before and change the water at least 5 times).

3. Bring to a boil briefly, in boiling water, for 5 minutes.

4. Crush the cod into chips, then.

5. In a frying pan, put ample oil and cook the onion and garlic. Then add 2 1/4 lb of boiled and squeezed potatoes 2 butter spoons 1/2 cup of milk Salt to taste Sour cream and bell peppers and simmer for about 10 minutes.

6. Then add the cod and olives and let it simmer for 10 further minutes.

7. Without letting so much of it dry out. And, to taste, apply oregano. You don't usually have to add salt since the cod already contains plenty of it.

8. If you need to bring in a bit, however.

9. Play over mashed potatoes with this braised cod. Cream:: Cream

10. In a blender, beat all the ingredients and pour over the cod.

11. For 30 minutes or until it is orange, take it to the previously heated air fryer at 6000F.

12. Serve with a leafy salad and white rice.

69.Gratinated Cod with Vegetables

Preparation Time: 10 Minutes

Cooking Time: 30 Minutes

Servings: 2-4

Ingredients:

- 2 ¼ lb cod 1 pound of potato 1 pound carrot
- 2 large onions
- 2 red tomatoes
- 1 bell pepper

- 1 tbsp. of tomato paste
- Coconut milk
- Garlic, salt, coriander and olive oil to taste.
- Olives

Sauce:

1. For 24 hours, soak the cod, always changing the water. Blanch, removing skin and pimples, at a fast boil. Strain and reserve the water where the cod has been cooked.

2. Season the French fries with cod, garlic, salt and coriander. On top of that, put a saucepan with olive oil and sliced onions on the fire. Add the onions, pepper, and chopped olives, skinless and seedless. Mix in the cod, tomato extract, coconut milk, and a little water to prepare the cod. Let them all cook a lot. There was a lot of sauce moving on. Get the salt tested. Sliced potatoes and carrots are cooked.

3. In a blender, whisk together milk, wheat and 2 cups milk 1 1/2 tablespoons all-purpose flour 1 tablespoon butter 1 egg 1/2 cup sour cream Nutmeg, black pepper and melted salt butter. Bring it to the fire and stir until it thickens the mixture. Finally, add the milk, nutmeg, black pepper, beaten egg and salt.

4. After rubbing a clove of garlic inside, grease a plate with olive oil. In alternate layers, arrange the cod, potato, and carrot. Cover all with sauce and bake for 20 minutes in an air fryer at 3800F.

70.Salmon Fillet

Preparation Time: 10 Minutes

Cooking Time: 15 Minutes

Servings: 2-4

Ingredients:

- 1 lb salmon fillet
- Sliced pitted olives
- Oregano
- 3 tbsp. soy sauce
- Salt to taste
- Olive oil to taste
- Lemon
- Aluminum foil
- ½ sliced onion

Directions:

1. Wash the salmon with lemon juice.

2. Heat the oil and add the sliced onion, leaving it on the fire until it becomes transparent. Reservation.

3. Cover a baking sheet with aluminum foil so that leftovers can cover all the fish.

4. In the foil on the baking sheet, place the fish already seasoned with salt, drizzle with olive oil and soy sauce.

5. Garnish with sliced olives and a little oregano. Pour the onion on top. Wrap with aluminum foil so that the liquid does not spill when it starts to heat up.

6. Bake in the air fryer at 4000F for about 30 minutes.

7. Serve with vegetables and green salad.

71.Hake Fillet with Potatoes
Preparation Time: 10 Minutes

Cooking Time: 30 Minutes

Servings: 2-4

Ingredients:

- 8 fillets of hake

- 4 raw potatoes
- 1 bell pepper
- 2 tomatoes
- 1 onion Good quality tomato sauce.
- Oregano
- Oil for greasing

Directions:

1. As desired, season the fillets and reserve for 10 minutes. Use olive oil to grease an ovenproof dish to create a coat of potato, then put the fillets on the potato. Drizzle with tomato sauce (1/2 can) and add onion, tomato, bell pepper, oregano to taste.

2. With the rest of the potatoes, seal. Cover and bake with foil until the potatoes are tender. Using lemon juice, wash the salmon. Heat the oil until it becomes transparent, and add the sliced onion, leaving it on the flames. On reservation.

3. Cover a baking sheet of aluminum foil so that all the fish can be covered with leftovers.

4. Place the fish, which is already seasoned with salt in the foil on the baking sheet, drizzle with olive oil and soy sauce.

5. Add chopped olives and a little oregano to the garnish. On top, pour the onion. Wrap the aluminum foil so that as it begins to heat up, the liquid does not leak.

6. Bake in an air-fryer for about 30 minutes at 4000F. 7. Serve with green salad and vegetables.

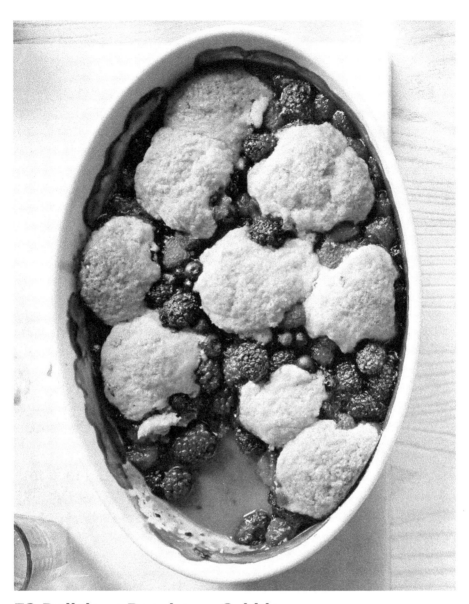

72.Delicious Raspberry Cobbler

Total time: 20 min

Prep time: 10 min

Cook time: 10 min

Yield: 6 serving

Ingredients:

- 1 egg, lightly beaten
- 1 cup raspberries, sliced
- 2 tsp. swerve
- 1/2 tsp. vanilla
- 1 tbsp. butter, melted
- 1 cup almond flour

Directions:

1. Place the Cuisinart oven in place 1. With the rack.
2. To the baking dish, add the raspberries.
3. Sprinkle with raspberries and sweetener.
4. In a dish, combine the almond flour, vanilla, and butter together.
5. Apply the egg to the mixture of almond flour and whisk well to blend.
6. Spread a mixture of almond flour over the sliced raspberries.
7. Set for 15 minutes to bake at 350 f. Place the baking dish in the preheated oven after five minutes.
8. Enjoy and serve.

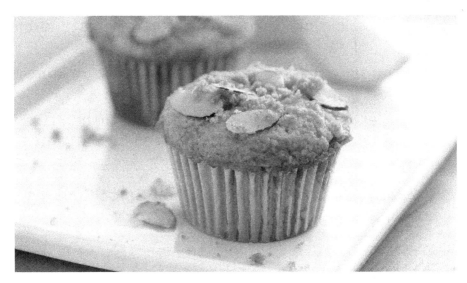

73.Orange Almond Muffins

Total time: 30 min

Prep time: 10 min

Cook time: 25 min

Yield: 2 servings

Ingredients:

- 4 eggs
- 1 tsp. baking soda
- 1 orange zest
- 1 orange juice
- 1/2 cup butter, melted
- 3 cups almond flour

Directions:

1. Place the Cuisinart oven in place 1. with the rack.
2. Line and set aside 12-cups of a muffin tin with cupcake liners.

3. In a big bowl, add all the ingredients and blend until well mixed.

4. In the prepared muffin pan, pour the mixture into it.

5. Set for 25 minutes to bake at 350 f. Place the muffin tin in the preheated oven for 5 minutes.

6. Enjoy and serve.

74. Easy Almond Butter Pumpkin Spice Cookies

Total time: 30 min

Prep time: 10 min

Cook time: 25 min

Yield: 6 servings

Ingredients:

- 1/4 tsp. pumpkin pie spice
- 1 tsp. liquid Stevie
- 6 oz. almond butter
- 1/3 cup pumpkin puree

Directions:

1. Place the Cuisinart oven in place 1. with the rack.

2. In the food processor, add all ingredients and process until simply combined.

3. Into the parchment-lined baking tray, drop spoonsful of mixture.

4. Set to bake for 23 minutes at 350 f. Place the baking pan in the preheated oven after five minutes.

5. Enjoy and serve.

75. Moist Pound Cake

Total time: 40 min

Prep time: 15 min

Cook time: 25 min

Yield: 2 serving

Ingredients:

- 4 eggs
- 1 cup almond flour
- 1/2 cup sour cream
- 1 tsp. vanilla
- 1 cup monk fruit sweetener
- 1/4 cup cream cheese
- 1/4 cup butter
- 1 tsp. baking powder
- 1 tbsp. coconut flour

Directions:

1. Place the Cuisinart oven in place 1. With the rack.
2. Mix the almond flour, baking powder, and coconut flour together in a big bowl.
3. Add the cream cheese and butter to a separate bowl and microwave for 30 seconds. Stir well, then microwave for 30 more seconds.
4. Stir in the sour cream, sweetener, and vanilla. Only stir well.
5. Pour the mixture of cream cheese into the almond flour mixture and whisk until mixed.
6. Add the eggs one by one to the batter and stir until well mixed.
7. Pour the batter into a cake pan of prepared oil.

8. Set to bake for 60 minutes at 350 f. Place the cake pans in the preheated oven after five minutes.

9. Slicing and serving.

76. Banana Butter Brownie

Total time: 25 min

Prep time: 10 min

Cook time: 15 min

Yield: 6 serving

Ingredients:

- 1 scoop protein powder
- 2 tbsp. cocoa powder
- 1 cup bananas, overripe
- 1/2 cup almond butter, melted

Directions:

1. Place the Cuisinart oven in place 1. with the rack.
2. In the blender, add all the ingredients and blend until smooth.
3. Fill the greased cake pan with batter.
4. Set for 21 minutes to bake at 325 f. Place the cake pans in the preheated oven after five minutes.
5. Enjoy and serve.

77. Peanut Butter Muffins

Total time: 10 min

Prep time: 15 min

Cook time: 15 min

Yield: 12 serving

Ingredients:

- 1 cup peanut butter
- 1/2 cup maple syrup
- 1/2 cup of cocoa powder
- 1 cup applesauce
- 1 tsp. baking soda
- 1 tsp. vanilla

Directions:

1. Place the Cuisinart oven in place 1. with the rack.
2. Line and set aside 12-cups of a muffin tin with cupcake liners.
3. In the blender, add all the ingredients and blend until smooth.
4. Pour the blended mixture into the muffin tin you have packed.
5. Set for 25 minutes to bake at 350 f. Place the muffin tin in the preheated oven for 5 minutes.
6. Enjoy and serve.

78.Baked Apple Slices

Total time: 40 min

Prep time: 15 min

Cook time: 25 min

Yield: 6 serving

Ingredients:

- 2 apples, peel, core, and slice
- 1 tsp. cinnamon
- 2 tbsp. butter
- 1/4 cup of sugar
- 1/4 cup brown sugar

- 1/4 tsp. salt

Directions:

1. Place the Cuisinart oven in place 1. with the rack.
2. In the zip-lock container, add cinnamon, sugar, brown sugar, and salt and combine well.
3. Fill the bag with apple slices and shake until well coated.
4. Apply the apple slices to the greased 9-inch baking dish.
5. Set to bake for 35 minutes at 350 f. Place the baking dish in the preheated oven after five minutes.
6. Enjoy and serve.

79.Vanilla Peanut Butter Cake

Total time: 40 min

Prep time: 15 min

Cook time: 25 min

Yield: 8 serving

Ingredients:

- 1 1/2 cups all-purpose flour
- 1/3 cup vegetable oil
- 1 tsp. baking soda
- 1/2 cup peanut butter powder
- 1 tsp. vanilla
- 1 tbsp. apple cider vinegar
- 1 cup of water
- 1 cup of sugar
- 1/2 tsp. salt

Directions:

1. Place the Cuisinart oven in place 1. with the rack.
2. Mix the flour, baking soda, peanut butter powder, sugar and salt together in a large mixing bowl.
3. Whisk the oil, vanilla, vinegar, and water together in a small cup.
4. Pour the mixture of oil into the mixture of flour and whisk until well mixed.
5. Fill the greased cake pan with batter.
6. Set to bake for 35 minutes at 350 f. Place the cake pans in the preheated oven after five minutes
7. Cut and serve.

80.Moist Chocolate Brownies

Total time: 25 min

Prep time: 10 min

Cook time: 15 min

Yield: 6 serving

Ingredients:

- 1 1/3 cups all-purpose flour
- 1/2 tsp. baking powder
- 1/3 cup cocoa powder
- 1 cup of sugar
- 1/2 tsp. vanilla
- 1/2 cup vegetable oil
- 1/2 cup water
- 1/2 tsp. salt

Directions:

1. Place the cuisine-style oven with the rack in place 1.

2. Mix the flour, baking powder, cocoa powder, sugar and salt together in a large mixing bowl.

3. Whisk the oil, water and vanilla together in a small cup.

4. Pour the mixture of oil into the flour and blend until well mixed.

5. Pour in the greased baking dish with the batter.

6. Set to bake for 25 minutes at 350 f. Place the baking sheet in the preheated oven after five minutes.

7. Cut and serve.

81.Yummy Scalloped Pineapple

Total time: 40 min

Prep time: 10 min

Cook time: 25 min

Yield: 6 serving

Ingredients:

- 3 eggs, lightly beaten
- 8 oz. can crush pineapple, un-drained
- 2 cups of sugar
- 4 cups of bread cubes
- 1/4 cup milk
- 1/2 cup butter, melted

Directions:

1. Place the Cuisinart oven in place 1. with the rack.

2. Mix the eggs with the milk, butter, crushed pineapple, and sugar in a mixing cup.

3. To coat, add bread cubes and stir well.

4. Move the mixture to a greased dish for baking.

5. Set to bake for 40 minutes at 350 f. Place the baking dish in the preheated oven after five minutes.

6. Enjoy and serve.

82.Vanilla Lemon Cupcakes

Total time: 25 min

Prep time: 10 min

Cook time: 15 min

Yield: 6 serving

Ingredients:

- 1 egg
- 1/2 cup milk
- 2 tbsp. canola oil
- 1/4 tsp. baking soda
- 3/4 tsp. baking powder
- 1 tsp. lemon zest, grated
- 1/2 cup sugar
- 1 cup flour
- 1/2 tsp. vanilla
- 1/2 tsp. salt

Directions:

1. Place the Cuisinart oven in place 1. with the rack.

2. Line and set aside 12-cups of a muffin tin with cupcake liners.

3. Whisk the egg, vanilla, milk, oil, and sugar together in a bowl until smooth.

4. Apply the remaining ingredients and combine until mixed.

5. Load the batter into the muffin tin that has been packed.

6. Set for 20 minutes to bake at 350 f. Place the muffin tin in the preheated oven for 5 minutes.

7. Enjoy and serve.

83. Walnut Carrot Cake

Total time: 25 min

Prep time: 10 min

Cook time: 15 min

Yield: 4 serving

Ingredients:

- 1 egg
- 1/2 cup sugar
- 1/4 cup canola oil
- 1/4 cup walnuts, chopped
- 1/2 tsp. baking powder
- 1/2 cup flour
- 1/4 cup grated carrot
- 1/2 tsp. vanilla
- 1/2 tsp. cinnamon

Directions:

1. Place the Cuisinart oven in place 1. with the rack.

2. Beat the sugar and oil in a medium bowl for 1 minute. Apply the vanilla, egg and cinnamon and beat for 30 seconds.

3. Apply the remaining ingredients and stir well until mixed.

4. Pour the batter into the baking bowl, which is greased.

5. Set for 30 minutes to bake at 350 f. Place the baking dish in the preheated oven after five minutes.

6. Enjoy and serve.

84.Baked Peaches

Total time: 40 min

Prep time: 10 min

Cook time: 25 min

Yield: 6 serving

Ingredients:

- 4 freestone peaches, cut in half and remove stones
- 2 tbsp. sugar
- 8 tsp. brown sugar
- 1 tsp. cinnamon
- 4 tbsp. butter, cut into pieces

Directions:

1. Place the Cuisinart oven in place 1. with the rack.

2. In a baking dish, put the peach halves and fill each half with 1 tsp. of brown sugar.

3. Place butter on top of the halves of each peach.

4. Mix the cinnamon and sugar together and drizzle over the peaches.

5. Set for 30 minutes to bake at 375 f. Place the baking dish in the preheated oven after five minutes.

6. Enjoy and serve.

85.Cinnamon Apple Crisp

Total time: 35 min

Prep time: 10 min

Cook time: 20 min

Yield: 4 serving

Ingredients:

- 1/8 tsp. ground clove
- 1/8 tsp. ground nutmeg
- 2 tbsp. honey
- 4 1/2 cups apples, diced
- 1 tsp. ground cinnamon
- 1 tbsp. cornstarch
- 1 tsp. vanilla
- 1/2 lemon juice
- For topping:
- 1 cup rolled oats
- 1/3 cup coconut oil, melted
- 1 tsp. cinnamon
- 1/3 cup honey
- 1/2 cup almond flour

Directions:

1. Place the Cuisinart oven in place 1. with the rack.

2. Mix the apples, vanilla, lemon juice, and honey in a medium-sized dish. Sprinkle it on top of herbs and cornstarch and stir well.

3. Load the combination of apples into the greased baking bowl.

4. Mix together the coconut oil, cinnamon, almond flour, oats and honey in a small bowl and scatter over the apple mixture.

5. Set to bake for 40 minutes at 350 f. Place the baking dish in the preheated oven after five minutes.

6. Enjoy and serve.

86.Apple Cake

Total time: 35 min

Prep time: 15 min

Cook time: 20 min

Yield: 12 serving

Ingredients:

- 2 cups apples, peeled and chopped
- 1/4 cup sugar
- 1/4 cup butter, melted
- 12 oz. apple juice
- 3 cups all-purpose flour
- 3 tsp. baking powder
- 1 1/2 tbsp. ground cinnamon
- 1 tsp. salt

Directions:

1. Place the Cuisinart oven in place 1. with the rack.
2. Mix the rice, salt, sugar, cinnamon, and baking powder together in a big dish.
3. Mix until well mixed, add melted butter and apple juice and mix.
4. Attach apples and fold thoroughly.
5. Pour the batter into the baking bowl, which is greased.
6. Set for 45 minutes to bake at 350 f. Place the baking dish in the preheated oven after five minutes.
7. Enjoy and serve.

87. Almond Cranberry Muffins

Total time: 35 min

Prep time: 15 min

Cook time: 20 min

Yield: 6 serving

Ingredients:

- 2 eggs
- 1 tsp. vanilla
- 1/4 cup sour cream
- 1/2 cup cranberries
- 1 1/2 cups almond flour
- 1/4 tsp. cinnamon
- 1 tsp. baking powder
- 1/4 cup swerve
- Pinch of salt

Directions:

1. Place the Cuisinart oven in place 1. with the rack.
2. Set aside and line 6-cups of a muffin tin with cupcake liners.
3. Put the sour cream, vanilla, and eggs in a cup.
4. Attach the remaining ingredients and beat until smooth, save for the cranberries.
5. Remove cranberries and fold thoroughly.
6. Load the batter into the muffin tin that has been packed.
7. Set for 30 minutes to bake at 325 f. Place the muffin tin in the preheated oven for 5 minutes.
8. Enjoy and serve.

88.Vanilla Butter Cake

Total time: 30 min

Prep time: 10 min

Cook time: 20 min

Yield: 8 serving

Ingredients:

- 1 egg, beaten
- 1/2 tsp. vanilla
- 3/4 cup sugar
- 1 cup all-purpose flour
- 1/2 cup butter, softened

Directions:

1. Place the cuisine-style oven with the rack in place 1.
2. Mix the sugar and butter together in a mixing cup.

3. Apply the egg, rice, and vanilla and whisk until mixed together.

4. Pour in the greased baking dish with the batter.

5. Set for 35 minutes to bake at 350 f. Place the baking sheet in the preheated oven after five minutes.

6. Cut and eat.

89.Coconut Butter Apple Bars

Total time: 40 min

Prep time: 10 min

Cook time: 30 min

Yield: 8 serving

Ingredients:

- 1 tbsp. ground flax seed
- 1/4 cup coconut butter, softened
- 1 cup pecans
- 1 cup of water
- 1/4 cup dried apples
- 1 1/2 tsp. baking powder
- 1 1/2 tsp. cinnamon
- 1 tsp. vanilla
- 2 tbsp. swerve

Directions:

1. Place the cuisine-style oven with the rack in place 1.

2. In the blender, add all of the ingredients and blend until smooth.

3. Pour the mixed mixture into the baking dish with oil.

4. Set to bake for 50 minutes at 350 f. Place the baking sheet in the preheated oven after five minutes.

5. Cut and eat.

90.Easy Blueberry Muffins

Total time: 40 min

Prep time: 10 min

Cook time: 30 min

Yield: 8 serving

Ingredients:

- o   oz. plain yogurt
- ½ cup fresh blueberries
- 2 tsp. baking powder, gluten-free
- ¼ cup swerve
- 2 ½ cups almond flour
- ½ tsp. vanilla
- 3 eggs
- Pinch of salt

Directions:

1. Place the Cuisinart oven in place 1. with the rack.

2. Set aside and line 6-cups of a muffin tin with cupcake liners.

3. Mix the egg, yogurt, vanilla, and salt in a bowl until smooth.

4. Add the flour, swerve and baking powder, and mix until smooth again.

5. Add the blueberries and blend well with them.

6. Load the batter into the muffin tin that has been packed.

7. Placed to bake for 35 minutes at 325 f. Place the muffin tin in the preheated oven for 5 minutes.

8. Enjoy and serve.

91. Tasty Almond Macaroons

Total time: 20 min

Prep time: 10 min

Cook time: 10 min

Yield: 12 serving

Ingredients:

- 2 egg whites
- 10 oz. almonds, sliced
- 1/2 tsp. vanilla extract
- 3/4 cup Splenda

Directions:

1. Place the Cuisinart oven in place 1. with the rack.

2. Beat the egg whites in a bowl until foamy, then add the Splenda and vanilla and mix until low.

3. Apply the egg mixture to the almonds and fold softly.

4. Slip the mixture into the parchment-lined baking pan using a spoon.

5. Set for 15 minutes to bake at 350 f. Place the baking pan in the preheated oven after five minutes.

6. Enjoy and serve.

92.Moist Baked Donuts

Total time: 20 min

Prep time: 10 min

Cook time: 10 min

Yield: 12 serving

Ingredients:

- 2 eggs
- 3/4 cup sugar
- 1/2 cup buttermilk
- 1/4 cup vegetable oil
- 1 cup all-purpose flour
- 1/2 tsp. vanilla
- 1 tsp. baking powder
- 1/2 tsp. salt

Directions:

1. Place the Cuisinart oven in place 1. with the rack.
2. Spray the donut pan and set it aside with the cooking spray.
3. Mix the oil, vanilla, baking powder, sugar, eggs, buttermilk, and salt together in a bowl until well mixed.
4. Stir in the flour and blend until the mixture is tender.
5. Load the batter into the donut pan that has been packed.
6. Set for 20 minutes to bake at 350 f. Place the donut pans in the preheated oven after five minutes.
7. Enjoy and serve.

93.Eggless Brownies

Total time: 40 min

Prep time: 10 min

Cook time: 30 min

Yield: 12 serving

Ingredients:

- 1/4 cup walnuts, chopped
- 1/3 cup cocoa powder
- 2 tsp. baking powder
- 1 cup of sugar
- 1 cup all-purpose flour
- 1/2 cup chocolate chips
- 2 tsp. vanilla
- 1 tbsp. milk
- 3/4 cup yogurt
- 1/2 cup butter, melted
- 1/4 tsp. salt

Directions:

1. Place the cuisine-style oven with the rack in place 1.

2. Sift the rice, chocolate powder, baking powder and salt into a large mixing cup. Mix and put aside well.

3. Add the sugar, vanilla, cream, and yogurt to another dish, and whisk until well mixed.

4. Apply the flour mixture to the mixture of butter and combine until just blended.

5. Fold in some chocolate chips and walnuts.

6. Pour the batter into a baking dish that has been packed.

7. Set to bake for 45 minutes at 350 f. Place the baking sheet in the preheated oven after five minutes.

8. Cut and eat.

94.Vanilla Banana Brownies

Total time: 40 min

Prep time: 10 min

Cook time: 30 min

Yield: 12 serving

Ingredients:

- 1 egg
- 1 cup all-purpose flour
- 4 oz. white chocolate
- 1/4 cup butter
- 1 tsp. vanilla extract
- 1/2 cup granulated sugar
- 2 medium bananas, mashed
- 1/4 tsp. salt

Directions:

1. Place the cuisine-style oven with the rack in place 1.

2. In a microwave-safe mug, add white chocolate and butter, and microwave for 30 seconds. Stir until it melts.

3. Send sugar a stir. Add mashed bananas, vanilla, eggs, and salt and combine until mixed together.

4. Attach rice, then blend until just blended together.

5. Pour in the greased baking dish with the batter.

6. Placed to bake for 25 minutes at 350 f. Place the baking sheet in the preheated oven after five minutes.

7. Cut and eat.

95.Choco Cookies

Total time: 20 min

Prep time: 10 min

Cook time: 10 min

Yield: 12 serving

Ingredients:

- 3 egg whites
- 3/4 cup cocoa powder, unsweetened
- 1 3/4 cup confectioner sugar
- 1 1/2 tsp. vanilla

Directions:

1. Place the Cuisinart oven in place 1. with the rack.

2. Whip the egg whites in a mixing bowl until the soft peaks are fluffy. Add the chocolate, cinnamon, and vanilla slowly.

3. Drop the teaspoonful into 32 tiny cookies on a parchment-lined baking pan.

4. Set for 8 minutes to bake at 350 f. Place the baking pan in the preheated oven after five minutes.

5. Enjoy and serve.

96.Chocolate Chip Cookies

Total time: 20 min

Prep time: 10 min

Cook time: 10 min

Yield: 30 serving

Ingredients:

- 1 egg
- 2/3 cup sugar
- 1 tsp. vanilla
- 1 cup butter, softened
- 12 oz. chocolate chips
- 2 cups self-rising flour
- 1/2 cup brown sugar

Directions:

1. Place the Cuisinart oven in place 1. with the rack.
2. In a broad mixing cup, add the sugar, vanilla, and egg and beat until mixed.
3. Apply the brown sugar and sugar and mix until smooth.
4. Add the flour slowly and stir until just mixed.
5. Fold the chocolate chips together.
6. Spoon the cookie dough balls into a baking tray lined with parchment.
7. Set for 15 minutes to bake at 375 f. Place the baking pan in the preheated oven after five minutes.
8. Enjoy and serve.

97.Oatmeal Cake

Total time: 40 min

Prep time: 10 min

Cook time: 30 min

Yield: 8 serving

Ingredients:

- 2 eggs, beaten
- 1 tbsp. cocoa powder
- 1/2 tsp. salt
- 1 tsp. baking soda
- 1/2 cup butter, softened
- 1 cup granulated sugar
- 1 cup brown sugar
- 1 3/4 cups flour
- 1 cup quick oats
- 3/4 cup mix nuts, chopped
- 2 cups chocolate chips
- 1 3/4 cup boiling water

Directions:

1. Place the cuisine-style oven with the rack in place 1.
2. Combine the boiling water in a large bowl with the oats.
3. Stir in the butter and sugar before the butter has melted.
4. Combine the rice, baking soda, cinnamon, cocoa powder, 1 cup of chocolate chips, half the diced nuts, and the egg. Mix once combined.
5. Sprinkle the remaining nuts and chocolate chips over the top of the cake batter and add the batter into the greased cake tin.

6. Set to bake for 45 minutes at 350 f. Place the baking sheet in the preheated oven after five minutes.

7. Cut and eat.

98.Delicious Banana Cake

Total time: 50 min

Prep time: 10 min

Cook time: 40 min

Yield: 8 serving

Ingredients:

- 2 large eggs, beaten
- 1 tsp. baking powder
- 1 1/2 cup sugar, granulated
- 1 tsp. vanilla extract
- 1/2 cup butter
- 1 cup milk
- 2 cups all-purpose flour
- 2 bananas, mashed
- 1 tsp. baking soda

Directions:

1. Place the cuisine-style oven with the rack in place 1.

2. Beat the sugar and butter together in a mixing bowl until smooth. Beaten eggs are inserted to blend properly.

3. Apply to the mixture the milk, vanilla extract, baking soda, baking powder, flour, and mashed bananas, and beat for 2 minutes. Mix thoroughly.

4. Pour in the greased baking dish with the batter.

5. Set to bake for 45 minutes at 350 f. Place the baking sheet in the preheated oven after five minutes.

6. Slice and eat.

99.Chocolate Cake

Total time: 50 min

Prep time: 10 min

Cook time: 40 min

Yield: 8 serving

Ingredients:

- 1/2 cup warm water
- 2 3/4 cups flour
- 1 cup buttermilk
- 1 cup shortening
- 1 cup sugar, granulated
- 1 cup brown sugar
- 2 large eggs
- 1/2 cup cocoa powder
- 1 tsp. baking soda

Directions:

1. Place the cuisine-style oven with the rack in place 1.

2. Beat together powdered sugar, granulated sugar and shortening until smooth in a large mixing cup.

3. Mix well with the eggs, cocoa powder, rice, and buttermilk when combined.

4. In warm water, dissolve the soda and stir into the batter.

5. Pour in the greased baking dish with the batter.

6. Set for 35 minutes to bake at 350 f. Place the baking sheet in the preheated oven after five minutes.

7. Slice and eat.

100.Almond Blueberry Bars

Total time: 60 min

Prep time: 10 min

Cook time: 40 min

Yield: 8 serving

Ingredients:

- 1/4 cup blueberries
- 3 tbsp. coconut oil
- 2 tbsp. coconut flour
- 1/2 cup almond flour
- 3 tbsp. water
- 1 tbsp. chia seeds
- 1 tsp. vanilla
- 1 tsp. fresh lemon juice
- 2 tbsp. erythritol
- 1/4 cup almonds, sliced
- 1/4 cup coconut flakes

Directions:

1. Place the Cuisinart oven with the rack in place 1.

2. Line a baking dish and set it aside with parchment paper.

3. Mix the water and the chia seeds together in a shallow cup. Put back aside.

4. In a tub, mix all of the ingredients together. Attach a blend of chia and whisk well.

5. Pour the mixture into the baking dish prepared and spread uniformly.

6. Set to bake for 55 minutes, at 300 f. Place the baking dish in the preheated oven after five minutes.

7. Slice and eat.

Conclusion

What is so unique about air frying, though? In a fraction of the time, the air fryer will replace your refrigerator, your fridge, your deep fryer, and your dehydrator, and cook tasty meals uniformly. The air fryer is a game changer if you're trying to supply your family with nutritious meals, just don't have a lot of time. This book is a compilation of 100 amazing and palatable air fryer recipes that you must give a try.

THE CARNIVORE DIET

A BEGINNERS GUIDE TO CARNIVORE DIET; HOW TO START,MAIN BENEFITS AND MORE ..

Introduction:

The Carnivore Diet builds entirely of meat and animal products, excluding all other foods. It's called to help weight loss, temperament issues, and blood sugar guideline, among other medical problems. However, the diet is highly restrictive and likely unhealthy in the long term. Plus, no research backs its purported benefits.

While there's no authority significance of flesh carnivore diet, think about the carnivore diet as an eating regimen that covers "just food varieties that strolled, swam, or flew," says Kelly Schmidt, RD, a holistic dietitian in personal exercise in Columbus, Ohio. While it may be a trend, "eating only meat is not hot. It's not colorful, and it's not fun," she says, adding that people who follow it do so because of a dynamic, motivating measure. Often that's to try to address an autoimmune salvo or try to lose weight.

The carnivore diet is often a rule people take after trying the paleo diet or the ketogenic diet, says Diana Rodgers, RD, of the Sustainable Dish, who lived in Concord, Massachusetts. Paleo or the "caveman" diet navels on fresh fruits, vegetables, grass-fed meats, and wild seafood whilst eliminating added sugars, grains, dairy, and legumes.

The Carnivore Diet is a master diet regimen that incorporates meat, fish, and other creature food varieties like eggs and specific dairy. It crops all other foods, including fruits, vegetables, legumes, grains, nuts, and seeds. Its proponents also consult eliminating or limiting dairy intake to foods based on lactose — a sugar establishes in milk and dairy manufactures — such as butter and solid cheeses.

The Carnivore Diet stems from the agitated belief that human paternal populations usually ate meat and fish and that high-carb diets are to reproach today's high rates of chronic illness. Other exoteric low-carb diets, like the keto and paleo diets, boundary but don't trim carb intake—however, the Carnivore Diet destinations for empty carbs.

Shawn Baker, a former American orthopaedic doctor, is the more significant portion well-known proponent of the Carnivore Diet. He refers to tributes from the individuals who follow the Carnivore Diet as a standard that can treat dumps, tension, joint pain, bloatedness, diabetes, and that's only the tip of the iceberg.

However, no research has explored the offshoots of the Carnivore Diet.

What's more, in 2017, Baker's medical permit was revoked by the New Mexico Medical Board due to anxieties about his foresight.

You will eat creature food sources—no natural products. No vegetables. Be that as it may, every one of the burgers and rib-eye steaks you can get your paws on.

Of the multitude of patterns that buck ordinary sustenance guidance, the meat-eater diet may seem like the most extreme one yet. It's one thing to suggest cutting carbs (the ketogenic diet) or eating just plant food sources, yet to recommend that creature food sources are all you should be solid and that vegetables can be adverse to wellbeing is a monster punch in the face to all that we were instructed in school and all the new sustenance and wellbeing features.

Everybody realizes that meat is risky; particularly on the off chance you eat a great deal of it... correct? Furthermore, that you need at any rate five servings of products of the soil each day... Or isn't that right?

On nit examined the flesh-eater diet down to the marrow and discovered what befalls your body when you burn through creatures, and that's it. Here's our manual for eating meat, bones, and organs for better wellbeing. We have divided the Carnivore Diet into 3 chapters. Let's look at the chapters:

Chapter 1: Tier of Carnivore Diet

I have shared some Carnivore Diet Tier. Now we will see some Carnivore Diet Tier:

Tier 1: Carnivore ISH

Otherwise called "carnivore adjoining", this sort of eating accentuates creature food varieties, and devours these as most of the diet, yet permits some space for what I would think about the most un-poisonous plant food varieties. Starting with an enthusiasm for the way that creature food varieties address the most supplement rich wellsprings of bioavailable nutrients and minerals, these food varieties structure most of such a diet, maybe 80%-90%. These food sources may incorporate ruminant (hamburger, buffalo, and sheep) meat, poultry, fish, eggs and dairy for the individuals who endure them (see conversation beneath for more data on this subject). Notwithstanding these food varieties, "low poisonousness" plant food sources might be incorporated for flavour, inclination or surface/shading. I will repeat here that I see plant food varieties as "endurance food varieties" and don't accept they give remarkable supplements to people that we can't acquire from creatures. Besides, plants have heaps of poisons in them, a significant number of which have been confused as valuable for people, that bother the gut and the resistant framework.

I consider the entire to be a creature-based diet as the most essential diet that people will flourish with. There seems, by all accounts, to be some hereditary changeability in human reaction to proportions of creature fats, in any case, and there are uncommon instances of people who don't oxidize fats for fuel well. For the VAST dominant part of individuals, nonetheless, a creature based diet is an ideal establishment. Hereditary changeability additionally seems to become an integral factor with respect to which plant food sources a given individual will endure. In certain people, any measure of plant food varieties and dairy seem to trigger the invulnerable framework, prompting a resurgence of irritation and autoimmunity. In others, explicit plant food sources might be endured without clear negative impacts. This is an individual quirk and should be resolved on such a premise. For the reasons for this blog entry, notwithstanding, I will examine a couple of food sources that may be viewed as the "least harmful," and that could be added to a "carnivore-ish" diet. The comprehension here, obviously, will be that quite a bit of this will be special dependent on the person.

Which are the most un-harmful plant food sources? I by and large consider these the non-sweet foods grown from the ground things like olives, avocado, lettuces, cucumbers (without skin or seeds), and different squashes in this gathering. Squash, specifically, will have higher measures of starches and will intrude on endeavours toward ketosis if that is an objective. On the other side, for those keen on joining sugars into their diets preceding long, serious athletic endeavours, squash may be a decent choice for this. Evacuation of skin and seeds of the squash would almost certainly diminish lectins essentially for this situation.

What might be said about more poisonous food varieties? At the furthest edge of the range, I would put plant seeds. The classification of plant seeds truly incorporates seeds, grains, nuts, and beans. These are all plant seeds, and they are largely vigorously guarded by plants. They contain stomach related compound inhibitors, lectins, high measures of physic corrosive an atom that ties phosphorus in plants yet can likewise tie other emphatically charged particles like Mg, Zn, Ca, and Se, restricting their assimilation. Notwithstanding plant seeds, the nightshade or Solanaceae family (tomatoes, eggplants, potatoes, goji berries, peppers, paprika, bean stew peppers) is likewise known to be a typical resistant trigger.

Most foods grown from the ground lie between these two gatherings and are hard to qualify as far as harmfulness. This will change from an individual to an individual premise. On a tier 1 Carnivore diet, you may begin with the low harmfulness plants and include moderate poisonousness food sources to perceive how you endure them. Numerous individuals will do best without any plants for some measure of time, nonetheless. At the point when all plants are dispensed, we move to a Tier 2 carnivore diet.

Refreshments: Many individuals get some information about espresso. I'll do an entirely separate post on this theme. The short answer is that I am not a devotee of espresso for an assortment of reasons including caffeine (thoughtful sensory system initiation, rest aggravation, and so forth), pesticides, shape poisons and acrylamide framed in the cooking interaction. In the event that you decide to remember espresso for your diet, realize that my overall experience is that the vast majority feel greatly improved without it whenever they have gone through the intense withdrawal stage. Instead of espresso, I by and large suggest superior grade, filtered water. Refined water or Reverse Osmosis ought to be demineralized yet is a decent alternative. Great carbon channels like the Berkey (no association) are another choice. The ideal water would be privately sourced spring water (findaspring.com), however, this isn't generally accessible. Shimmering mineral water is fine – I'm a major fanatic of Gerolsteiner, which is especially plentiful in minerals, and Topo Chico. Tea contains numerous mixtures, similar to tannins, which may impede supplement ingestion and bother the gut. I by and large advise against it. Soft drinks, organic product juices, and so forth are plainly not ideal and ought to have stayed away from.

Tier 2: Meat/Water

This is the most fundamental and least difficult rendition of a genuine carnivore diet. It's for individuals who need to explore different avenues regarding an entire food sources creature based diet for short measures of time, similar to an end diet. As I would like to think, this kind of carnivore eating isn't ideal for the vast majority in the long haul, yet it could fill in as a basic prologue to this method of eating.

On a Tier 2 Carnivore diet "eat meat, drink water" is the exemplary proverb that depicts this method of eating best. It's a beautiful basic recipe, and as a disposal diet, it tends to be an exceptionally supportive apparatus. My interests with this sort of diet long haul are supplement inadequacies. I did a digital broadcast with Amber O'Hearn wherein we discussed subtleties in regards to RDAs on a carnivore diet. It's quite certain that our body's necessities for some, things changes without starches. Indeed, even meat has few carbs however for the reasons for this conversation, they are basically insignificant. There's an entire Facebook bunch (Zeroing in on Health) committed to this sort of diet, and there are numerous instances of individuals who seem to flourish eating just creature meat and drinking water. Models incorporate Joe and Charlene Andersen, and Charles Washington, who directs the previously mentioned Facebook bunch.

While I do think a tier 2 carnivore diet can be extremely useful for certain individuals, adding even a couple of food varieties like eggs and periodic fish can help fill in a considerable lot of the expected supplement holes. Developmentally, I additionally don't believe that we would have just eaten the muscle meat of creatures. There are various models from anthropological writing to propose that numerous native people groups really preferred organ meats and fat, and ate muscle meat last, or even took care of the muscle meat to the canines. We'll speak more about adding organ meats in Tier 4/5 carnivore diets; above all, we should discuss adding only a couple more fundamental supplement rich creatures' food sources to the meat and water diet.

Tier 3: Basic Carnivore diet

The fundamental carnivore diet adds a couple of things to the Tier 2 Meat and Water plan. This where most people begin, and afterwards as the rule progress to Tiers 4 and 5 as they get more amped up for eating organ meats. The Tier 3 feast plan incorporates meat, eggs, fish, and dairy whenever endured.

A couple of words about dairy: I've actually tracked down that a wide range of dairy triggers my dermatitis, and in numerous customers, I work with, prohibition of dairy takes into account expanded satiety, less aggravation, and simpler weight reduction. As a rule, I do feel that dairy can be setting off for some individuals. On the off chance that you have an immune system issue or you are truly keen on getting more fit, I'd forget about dairy for in any event the initial 60 days of a Carnivore diet. There's a touch of subtlety here too with respect to A1 versus A2 variations of casein, what separates into beta casomorphin. The name of that particle resembles "morphine," and it acts in a comparable, however considerably less exceptional, route in the human body by initiating narcotic flagging pathways. I'll do an entirely separate blog entry about A1 versus A2 dairy. The precipice notes adaptation is that casein has two variations (quality polymorphisms, or SNPs), A1 and A2, which are separated into various types of beta-casomorphin.

The A1 variation of casein becomes beta-casomorphin 7, an atom that has been connected to the expanded frequency of immune system sickness and cardiovascular illness. The bring home message here is that in case you will do dairy and don't think it triggers your insusceptible framework, settle on A2 dairy as opposed to A1. All non-cow dairy including goat, sheep, and the wild ox is viewed as A2 dairy. There are cow-like species which are A2, in the same way as other Guernsey cows, yet these will be noted on the naming and are a lot more uncommon. In the event that it's from a cow and doesn't determine A2 on the mark, except that it's A1 dairy.

Tier 4: Junior varsity organ meat eating and real animal fats

This tier is for you in the event that you are cherishing the carnivore diet and are organ-inquisitive. You've heard me extoll the ideals of organ meats, similar to liver, and might want to fuse this into your diet.

You've likewise heard me talk about the astonishing ethics of grass-took care of fat decorations or suet (hamburger kidney fat) and you'd prefer to hop on the fat train. A tier 4 carnivore diet will presumably suit your requirements well indeed, and I accept that you will see enhancements in mental clearness, satiety, and athletic execution by updating your diet.

We should begin with the liver! Isn't this organ the body's channel and loaded with poisons? Probably not! The facts demonstrate that the liver contains most of the enzymatic frameworks associated with detoxification. These are alluded to as the stage 1 and stage 2 detox pathways. The liver doesn't store poisons, in any case. It artificially changes them with these frameworks to set up the poisons for EXCRETION in the pee and defecation. This is the means by which we dispose of the awful stuff – we don't need dreadful synthetic substances and mixtures sticking around our bodies. On the off chance that you've heard me talk about phytochemicals like sulforaphane or curcumin, you'll realize that these mixtures are detoxified in stage 1/2 and afterwards discharged. Indeed, I did surely call these mixtures poisons, and I don't feel they have any useful spot in human sustenance. You can discover substantially more inside and out conversations of plant poisons on a significant number of the web recordings I've been on. See the post on which digital broadcasts I've been on [here]. Especially the top bottom scene incorporates Peak Human and Ben Greenfield.

So the liver isn't a channel, you get it, yet you didn't grow up eating liver and the taste is not quite the same as what you are utilized to... Is it actually that particularly nutritious? In a word, yes! Muscle meat from creatures is plentiful in a ton of nutrients and minerals; however, it doesn't have every one of them. Basically adding liver to a Tier 3 carnivore diet truly helps fill in a considerable lot of the potential supplements that could be restricted on this kind of diet. Without a doubt, eating eggs and fish will give a larger number of supplements than a meat and water diet, yet I think including the liver will be far and away superior.

What supplements am I discussing here? The liver is especially plentiful in a couple of minerals and B nutrients which supplement those found in muscle meat. On the mineral side, the liver is probably the best wellspring of copper, which we need for catalysts like Super Oxide Dismutase (SOD). Turf serves a basic job in the cancer prevention agent the board framework in our bodies (I talk about this in the digital broadcast I did with Dom D'Agostino, PhD) by changing over the superoxide revolutionary (O2-) into sub-atomic oxygen (O2) or hydrogen peroxide (H2O2). A copper lack would bring about the gathering of O2-, which could have unfortunate outcomes as far as abundance oxidative pressure. Copper inadequacy is uncommon, yet it can happen in the event that we burn through a lot of zinc without some copper to adjust it. The most widely recognized circumstance for this to happen would be extreme utilization of zinc supplements without a decent wellspring of copper in our diets, however, it is likewise conceivable through diet in the event that we get a great deal of zinc in muscle meat without some wellspring of copper. Clinical copper lack shows with neurologic indications which impersonate B12 inadequacy (trouble with balance, strolling). Yowser! No good times!

Besides copper, the liver is likewise an extraordinary wellspring of MANY different minerals including iron, selenium, manganese, and molybdenum. It's likewise extremely wealthy in choline, which has been treacherously censured regarding TMAO (see the webcast I did with Tommy Wood, PhD in which we talk about this), and is a fundamental supplement for solid cell films and synapse creation.

Taking a gander at the B-nutrients, the liver is only a force to be reckoned with, on the request for the Incredible Hulk or other Avengers superhuman. It gives altogether more elevated levels of practically these supplements and is a particularly decent wellspring of folate, biotin, and riboflavin, which truly are not that accessible in muscle meat. In the event that you have an MTHFR or PEMT polymorphism (look at the webcast with Dr Ben Lynch), you'll require more riboflavin than everybody, and the liver is just about the most extravagant source there is! Other great wellsprings of riboflavin are heart, kidney, and egg yolks, with muscle meat having some however not close to as much as these uncommon food varieties. On the off chance that you are keen on eating heart and kidney, you are likely prepared for a Tier 5 Carnivore diet!

Tier 5: Optimal Nose to Tail Carnivore diet

You are centered on upgrading your diet for best outcomes regarding the goal of fiery issues, weight loss, or physical/mental execution, and you need the Ferrari variant of the carnivore diet. This is it! Tier 5 is fundamentally how I eat throughout each and every day. This is a definitive Carnivore MD diet. As I've noted before, this kind of carnivore diet may not be for everybody consistently. Voyaging makes eating loads of excellent creature meats, organs and fat troublesome every now and then, and I get this. It's absolutely alright to utilize Tier 1-4 diets in your day to day existence when they are the most suitable for your present circumstance. In these circumstances, parched organ enhancements can help make consolidating organ meats into your diet more advantageous.

So how would I eat, and what do I believe is the BEST method to develop a nose to tail carnivore diet? There several pieces to this condition. The primary thing I consider is the fat to protein proportion regarding macronutrients. I'll do an entirely separate post on this. On the off chance that you need to hear me out talking about the professionals/cons of high fat versus high protein with Ted Naiman, look at the Better, Stronger, Faster web recording I did with him here. I will likewise present a connection on my Ancestral Health discussion chat on the interesting supplement estimation of creature fat whenever it's posted.

My overall point of view is that creature fat is an imperative and significant piece of creatures that people have particularly searched out all through our reality, and which ought not to be ignored or underestimated. Very much like how the liver and the other organ meats have an interesting wholesome profile, creature fat does too and I accept that it ought to be purposefully remembered for an all-around developed nose to the tail carnivore diet. On the off chance that you are eating grass-took care of meat, there's some fat with cuts like ribeye and NY strip, however, it is anything but a ton. The vast majority of the fat is currently managed off our meat by butchers, so we need to explicitly request decorations or search for the fat around the kidneys (suet). Grain-took care of meat is absolutely fattier yet as I talk about in this blog entry, I have a few worries about grain-took care of fat aggregating more poisons like estrogen-imitating mixtures, pesticides and dioxins. By and by, I source grass-took care of suet from US Wellness Meats or White Oak Pastures (no alliance) and incorporate this as an enormous part of my diet.

What amount fat do I eat? Since I am at my objective bodyweight and organization, I am generally keen on athletic execution. In view of this, I focus on about 1.5-2g of fat per gram of protein that I eat consistently. For protein, I focus on about .8g per lb of fit bodyweight each day. As a 170 lb fella, this winds up being about 140g of protein and 230-280g of fat each day! Are these macros making me lose lean mass or collect fat? I'd say certainly not, however, I'll leave you alone the adjudicator.

The entirety of this grass-took care of creature fat I am devouring is a wellspring of remarkable supplements. What?! Does fat have supplements? Of course, it does! Grass-took care of creature fat is an incredible wellspring of fat-solvent nutrients like nutrient E and nutrient K2. In the Rotterdam Study, expanded utilization of nutrient K2, however, not K1 (from plants) was related with fundamentally improved coronary illness results. Grass-took care of creature fat is likewise a wellspring of the omega-3 unsaturated fats, EPA, DHA and DPA. My degrees of omega-3 are vigorous eating a tier 5 carnivore diet.

I additionally test my micronutrients, including nutrient E, consistently. The outcomes beneath are from July 2019. As should be obvious, my CoQ10 is off the graphs (this is basic in customers I work with on the carnivore diet), and my B nutrient markers are for the most part looking extraordinary. My homocysteine is 7, which is actually where I might want to see it. Strangely, I am homozygous for the 677C->T polymorphism of MTHFR, and I don't enhance with any methyl folate. It's obvious from this lab result that I am getting sufficient riboflavin from the liver I eat. The folate in the liver is likewise L-5 methyl folate, as opposed to dihydrofolate, as is found in plants. Look at the web recording I did with Dr Ben Lynch for a full conversation of these polymorphisms. I'll additionally do an entire digital broadcast and separate post pretty much the entirety of my blood work at last.

Seeing this part of my blood work, notice how high my nutrient E is. It's really over the reach True Health records as ordinary; however this is anything but something awful. I don't enhance with such a nutrient E. This is only coming from grass-took care of creature fat! One of the investigates that have been leveled against the carnivore diet is that this diet could be low in nutrient E. My outcomes, and the aftereffects of my customers, would contend emphatically against this. Look at the entire web recording I did noting regular evaluates of the carnivore diet in the event that you'd prefer to dive further into the entirety of this.

A tier 5 carnivore diet likewise incorporates loads of organ meats. I for one courtesy these in my diet and normally wind up eating an assortment of them for the duration of the day. I do attempt to turn the organ meats I eat over time as I accept our progenitors would have. What I accomplish may not work for everybody, and a portion of the organs I eat might be considered "net" regarding what is standard, yet I discover incredible worth in putting forth attempts to eat as a large part of the creature as possible. In a given week I will eat around 16 oz liver, 16 oz kidney, 16-32oz heart, 16oz balls, and intermittent spleen, pancreas, and cerebrum when they are free.

You absolutely don't need to eat these organs to do an extraordinary variant of a tier 5 carnivore diet, yet they merit investigating. This may likewise be where parched organ cases can assist us with getting a more extensive assortment of organs. In the part underneath about a regular tier 5 diet, I will depict what I eat so individuals can get a feeling of this. Once more, since I do it this way doesn't mean it's the best way to do it! The other disclaimer here is that while I eat numerous food sources crude, this surely presents defilement dangers and it's not something I suggest except if you know the nature of your sourcing quite well.

Chapter 2: Daily Food menu, Results and safety
Follow the Carnivore Diet

Following the Carnivore Diet includes eating just meat, fish, and creature items, taking out any remaining food sources. It gives no rules on calorie consumption, serving size, or supper timing. Following the diet includes disposing of all plant food varieties from your diet and solely eating meat, fish, eggs, and modest quantities of low-lactose dairy items. Food varieties to eat an incorporate hamburger, chicken, pork, sheep, turkey, organ meats, salmon, sardines, white fish, and limited quantities of weighty cream and hard cheddar. Spread, fat, and bone marrow are likewise permitted.

Defenders of the diet underscore eating greasy slices of meat to arrive at your day by day energy needs. The Carnivore Diet supports drinking water and bone stock however debilitate drinking tea, espresso, and different beverages produced using plants. It gives no particular rules with respect to calorie consumption, serving sizes, or the number of suppers or bites to eat each day. Most advocates of the diet propose eating as frequently as you want.

For individuals who wish to attempt the carnivore diet, here is a 5-day test menu:

Day 1

- **Breakfast:** Boiled eggs and bacon.
- **Lunch:** Chicken bosom or a Parmesan omelet.
- **Supper:** A hamburger burger patty with cut turkey and sharp cream.
- **Bites:** Beef jerky or sardines.

Day 2

- **Breakfast:** Scrambled eggs with spread.
- **Lunch:** A sheep burger with cheddar.
- **Supper:** Sausage, egg, and cheddar dish.
- **Bites:** Prawns or flame-broiled bacon cuts with Parmesan.

Day 3

- **Breakfast:** A chicken omelet.
- **Lunch:** A greasy cut of rib-eye steak or fried eggs.
- **Supper:** Fish with acrid cream or meat liver.
- **Tidbits:** A limited quantity of hard cheddar or bone stock.

Day 4

- **Breakfast:** Smoked salmon or squashed bubbled eggs.
- **Lunch:** Pork cleaves with nectar or a little glass of hefty cream.
- **Supper:** Beef meatballs or a cheddar omelet.
- **Bites:** Turkey jerky or bone marrow.

Day 5

- **Breakfast:** Turkey wieners with eggs.
- **Lunch:** Crab cooked in fat or scallops.
- **Supper:** Filet mignon or chicken liver.
- **Bites:** Chicken wings or bone stock.

Strict Carnivore Diet Food List
Allowed foods on this diet style include:

- All meat and fish
- Shellfish
- Poultry
- Eggs
- Organ meats
- Bone Marrow
- Bone Broth
- Jerky (no added sugar)
- Pork rinds
- Lard
- Tallow

Foods to avoid on this diet style include:

- Dairy: milk, yogurt, cheese, butter
- Fruits
- Vegetables
- Nuts and seeds
- Grains
- Processed foods
- Sugar
- Alcohol
- Tea and coffee
- Sweetened Beverages
- Vegetable oils

Standard Carnivore Diet Food List

A standard carnivore diet often allows for some high fat, low carb dairy products in addition.

Allowed foods on this diet style include:

- All meat and fish
- Shellfish
- Poultry
- Eggs
- Organ meats
- Bone marrow
- Bone broth
- Lard
- Tallow
- Pork rinds
- Jerky (no added sugar)
- High fat dairy: yogurt, butter, ghee cream, hard cheeses, kefir

Foods to avoid on this diet style include:

- Fruits
- Vegetables
- Nuts and seeds
- Grains
- Processed foods
- Sugar
- Alcohol
- Tea and coffee
- Sweetened Beverages
- Vegetable oils

Modified Carnivore Diet Food List

An adjusted carnivore diet approach will permit modest quantities of certain low sugar plant food varieties like avocado, lettuce, and cucumber.

Allowed foods on this diet style include:

- All meat and fish
- Shellfish
- Poultry
- Eggs
- Organ meats
- Bone marrow
- Bone broth
- Lard
- Tallow
- Pork rinds
- Jerky (no added sugar)
- Low carb dairy: yogurt, butter, ghee cream, cheese, kefir, cottage cheese
- Avocado
- Non-starchy veggies: cucumbers, lettuce, radish, celery, onion
- Tea and coffee
- Vegetable oils

Foods to avoid on this diet style include:

- Fruits
- Most Vegetables
- Nuts and seeds
- Grains
- Processed foods
- Sugar
- Alcohol
- Sweetened Beverages

Keto Carnivore Diet Food List

A keto carnivore diet permits marginally more plant food sources that are additionally keto diet affirmed, including certain nuts, seeds, and non-boring vegetables. Keto carnivore is basically a keto diet with more meat and fish accentuation.

Allowed foods on this diet style include:

- All meat and fish
- Shellfish
- Poultry
- Eggs
- Organ meats
- Bone marrow
- Bone broth
- Lard
- Tallow
- Pork rinds
- Jerky (no added sugar)
- Low carb dairy: yogurt, butter, ghee cream, cheese, kefir, cottage cheese
- Avocado
- Non-starchy veggies: cucumbers, lettuce, radish, celery, onion
- Nuts and seeds
- Tea and coffee
- Vegetable oils

Foods to avoid on this diet style include:

- Fruits
- Starchy Vegetables
- Grains
- Sugar
- Alcohol
- Sweetened Beverages

Sample Standard Carnivore Diet Food List

Thinking about what an all meat carnivore diet resembles practically speaking? Here's an example menu that one should seriously mull over eating when observing a standard carnivore diet.

Carnivore Diet Breakfast Options

- Eggs and sausage
- Shredded chicken and egg scramble
- Sardines and fried eggs

Carnivore Diet Lunch Options

- Tuna in oil and cheese slices
- Bun-less burger with cheese
- Chicken and sausage

Carnivore Diet Dinner Options

- Salmon and cream cheese
- Steak and shrimp
- Liver and cheese

Carnivore Diet Snack Options

- Hard-boiled eggs and sardines
- Jerky (no added sugar)
- Full fat yogurt
- Bone broth
- Kefir

The carnivore diet comprises creature food sources alone. However long the constituents of your dinner strolled, slithered, flew, swam, or in any case had guardians, they're reasonable game (no joke planned). You don't need to keep any principles to the extent of food timing, macronutrient breakdowns, or parts. Essentially eat when you're eager and until you're full. Coming up next are instances of endorsed carnivore diet food sources.

What if You Opt for Lean Meats, Like Fish and Poultry?

All things considered, you'd need to eat much more to arrive at a similar calorie level in case you're intending to zero in on lean poultry or fish decisions (like chicken bosom and cod). This may likewise keep you from going into ketosis, which is an objective of numerous individuals who go on extremely low or zero-carb diets. On the off chance that you need to be in ketosis, you'd need to decide on fattier meats as opposed to topping off on skinless chicken bosoms, yet once more, there is restricted exploration on how sound this is in general.

Meat

Steak, burgers, and red meat overall are the principal food hotspots for carnivore dieters. Since you're not eating carbs—or any plant food sources whatsoever—it's pivotal that you get enough calories to keep your energy up, so fattier cuts of meat are ideal. Poultry and organ meats are additionally fine, as are prepared meat items like bacon and wiener.

Fish

Any sort is OK, however, once more, fattier sorts, for example, salmon and sardines are the most intelligent decisions.

Entire Eggs

You'll require the fat in those yolks.

Dairy

Milk, cheddar, yogurt, and spread all come from creatures and are in fact allowable, albeit most carnivore dieters appear to preclude or if nothing else restrict them. This is ordinarily because of individuals finding the carnivore diet as an outgrowth of the ketogenic diet, in which milk and yogurt are by and large not allowed because of their lactose (sugar) content.

As one of the objectives of a carnivore diet is to dispose of supplements that your body will most likely be unable to measure ideally (see "Carnivore Diet Benefits"), you should try different things with dairy

146

food sources each in turn and in little portions to perceive how you handle them. You may discover you feel better with none by any means.

Bone Marrow

Bone broth is allowed.

Fatty Meat Products

Tallow, lard, and other fat-dense foods derived from meat are green lit.

Followers of the carnivore diet fluctuate in what they permit themselves to eat. The center standard of the diet is that an individual can just devour food varieties from creature sources. Toward one side of the range, a few groups eat one sort of meat in particular. At the opposite end, individuals incorporate an assortment of meat and certain dairy items in their diet. The accompanying areas will take a gander at which food varieties to incorporate and which food sources to stay away from.

Foods to eat

An individual after the carnivore diet may devour:

- Meat: like sheep, hamburger, chicken, turkey, pork, or organ meats
- Fish and fish: like salmon, mackerel, fish, sardines, herring, crab, or clams
- Other creature items: like eggs, bone stock, bone marrow, or grease
- Low lactose dairies: like spread, substantial cream, or hard cheddar like Parmesan
- Water

A few followers likewise devour salt, pepper, and different flavors that don't contain carbs. Nectar isn't permitted in an exacting carnivore diet; however, a few advocates incorporate it since it comes from a creature source, in spite of being high in glucose.

Any food varieties that don't come from creature sources are barred from the carnivore diet. These include:

- Fruits, such as bananas, berries, citrus fruits, apples, or avocado
- Vegetables, such as potatoes, carrots, broccoli, spinach, or peppers
- Grains, such as rice, wheat, bread, quinoa, cereals, or pasta
- Nuts and seeds, such as almonds, pecans, walnuts, pumpkin seeds, or sesame seeds
- High lactose dairies, such as soft cheese, milk, or yogurt
- Legumes, such as beans, lentils, peanuts, or soybeans
- Alcohol, such as wine, beer, or liquor
- Sugars, such as table sugar, brown sugar, maple syrup, or agave syrup
- Plant-based oils, such as sunflower oil, olive oil, coconut oil, or canola oil
- Beverages other than water, such as soda, tea, coffee, or fruit juice

Carnivore Diet Results: Will the Meal Plan Help With Weight Loss?

It may. You're eating only one kind of food — meat — so your calories will probably be more confined. For one, there's the satiety that this protein gives. At that point, there's the way that it wipes out careless eating, says Schmidt. "You don't carelessly eat chicken bosoms. It's an entirely satisfactory diet, however, you don't lick your plate," she says.

You may likewise go into a condition of ketosis on the carnivore diet, says Schmidt. Around there, your body is consuming fat for fuel as opposed to sugars. That is not an assurance, however. It's confusing that all you need is as far as possible carbs to get to ketosis — protein matters, as well.

"In abundance, protein can prompt an expansion in glucose and insulin levels, and it can show you out of ketosis," says Schmidt. Know your objectives. In the event that you will probably eat zero carbs, have simply meat. On the off chance that it's to be in ketosis, ensure that you center fundamentally around fattier wellsprings of meat, just as eggs and other fat sources, similar to cheddar and margarine.

Is The Carnivore Diet Safe?

Since it's like a ketogenic diet, and we've effectively shown that meat isn't at fault for coronary illness, it shows up reasonable to consider the carnivore diet ok for a great many people—in any event for the time being. Nonetheless, in the event that you've at any point seen the film Beverly Hills Cop, there's one inquiry you've been passing on to pose: is all that meat going to stall out in my gut?

In the film, one character peruses an (invented) article to another, referring to science that guarantees that "when the normal American is 50, he has five pounds of undigested red meat in his entrails." Based on this one scene in a well-known film from over 30 years prior—and an Eddie Murphy satire at that—the metropolitan legend has propagated that hamburger some way or another square up your digestive organs, colon... and so on.

Nonetheless, similarly, as you can't incapacitate a squad car by pushing a banana in its tailpipe (another piece of wacky science from the film), your body will not gag itself to death from eating rib-eyes.

"Like most food varieties, meat is invested in the small digestive organs before it arrives at the colon," says St. Pierre. "The possibility that meat gets affected in your GI plot is senseless." It's feasible to get a gut obstacle because of sickness or actual injury, "however red meat isn't something that impedes your GI parcel." Since there isn't a lot coming out, individuals who have little solid discharges will in general accept that waste is stalling out inside them. Yet, St. Pierre says that little developments, including those of carnivore dieters, are just because of low admissions of fiber. "Fiber adds mass," he says. So the explanation your crap is little is that it doesn't have veggies in it.

"I never had any distension, swelling, or water maintenance all through the entire cycle," says Munsey. "Truth be told, I felt light and had a skip in my progression."

A more genuine worry on the carnivore diet, nonetheless, is the danger of malignancy. "There's such a lot of proof on phytonutrients from plant food varieties and how they assist with DNA insurance," says St. Pierre. "In case you're not devouring those things, nobody's entirely certain regarding what that will mean for your long haul." Bacteria in the GI parcel and colon mature fiber into butyrate, a short-chain unsaturated fat. Butyrate diminishes irritation in the GI parcel, possibly diminishing the danger of colon malignancy.

"I would exceptionally presume that an all-creature diet would build your danger of colon malignancy," says St. Pierre. Not on the grounds, that creature food varieties are cancer-causing in any capacity, but since "you wouldn't be devouring things that help to restrain colon malignant growth. So the portion makes the toxin. Having a couple of servings of red meat every week is no biggie, yet when you're eating three steaks per day with nothing else, that is an alternate story. You're changing the condition considerably."

Also, eating leafy foods offer advantages for eye wellbeing, cerebrum wellbeing, and in general life span, says St. Pierre. "You'd disregard such a lot of exploration on their likely advantages by removing them all."

Another mainstream carnivore diet question: what befalls the gut biome? That is the equilibrium of microorganisms that help digest your food and forestall illness. Clearly, those critters should require some carbs. Or then again not.

"I had zero dysbiotic vegetation [the terrible bacteria] toward the finish of the diet," says Munsey, who had his crap tried. "What's more, I had very great numbers on all the gainful vegetation." He credits it to the carnivore diet being, if nothing else, a limited end diet that starves eager for sugar terrible microorganisms to death. "Better believe it, it would keep some from the great ones also, however perhaps we don't require as large numbers of those. Perhaps we possibly need them in

151

case we're eating a high-plant diet. It's rarely been examined, so for individuals to hop directly out and say the carnivore diet isn't right and terrible for your wellbeing... all things considered, we don't realize that."

Risks and side effects

The prohibitive idea of the carnivore diet avoids whole nutritional categories with regard to an individual's diet, accordingly barring the majority of the nutrients, minerals, and micronutrients they give. Vegetables, natural products, and grains contain fiber, which is fundamental for solid processing. Research Trusted Source has tracked down that dietary fiber can likewise secure against colon malignancy and colorectal adenoma.

As per some other research trusted Source, eating red meat and prepared meat is related to an expanded danger of coronary supply route sickness and diabetes. A further well-being hazard may originate from the kind of meat that an individual eats.

For instance, a few meats are high in immersed fat, which can bring cholesterol step up in the blood. Research Trusted Source has discovered that eating a ton of immersed fat over the long haul can expand an individual's danger of coronary illness.

For individuals with ongoing kidney sickness, following a high protein diet may be particularly harming.

Studies Trusted Source has proposed that restricting protein admission in individuals with CKD can moderate the movement of the condition and postpone the requirement for dialysis treatment. Restricting assortment in the diet could likewise be especially perilous for pregnant or lactating individuals, whose dietary requirements are probably not going to be met by an ASF diet.

Other disagreeable results of ASF and LCHF diets incorporate clogging, cerebral pains, awful breath, and fart.

Decadence of the Carnivore Diet

Because of its profoundly prohibitive nature and complete end of most nutrition classes, there are numerous disadvantages to the Carnivore Diet.

High in fat, cholesterol, and sodium

Given that the Carnivore Diet comprises exclusively of creature food sources, it very well may be high in immersed fat and cholesterol. Soaked fat may raise your LDL (terrible) cholesterol, which may expand your danger of coronary illness.

Nonetheless, late examinations have shown that high admissions of immersed fat and cholesterol are not emphatically connected to a higher danger of coronary illness, as was recently accepted. All things considered, devouring high measures of immersed fat on the Carnivore Diet might be of concern. No examination has broken down the impacts of eating creature food sources solely. Along these lines, the impacts of devouring such significant degrees of fat and cholesterol are obscure.

Additionally, some handled meats, particularly bacon and breakfast meats, likewise contain high measures of sodium. Eating a ton of these food varieties on the Carnivore Diet can prompt unnecessary sodium admission, which has been connected to an expanded danger of hypertension, kidney infection, and other negative wellbeing results. Handled meat consumption has likewise been connected to higher paces of specific sorts of malignant growth, including colon and rectal disease.

May come up short on specific micronutrients and valuable plant compounds

The Carnivore Diet dispenses with exceptionally nutritious food sources like organic products, vegetables, vegetables, and entire grains, all of which contain useful nutrients and minerals. While meat is nutritious and gives micronutrients, it ought not to be the solitary piece of your diet. Following a prohibitive diet like the Carnivore Diet may prompt lacks in certain supplements and the overconsumption of others.

In addition, diets that are wealthy in plant-based food sources have been related to a lower hazard of certain ongoing conditions like coronary illness, certain tumours, Alzheimer's, and type 2 diabetes. This isn't simply because of the great nutrient, fiber, and mineral substance of plant food varieties yet in addition their valuable plant mixtures and cancer prevention agents. The Carnivore Diet doesn't contain these mixtures and has not been related with any drawn out medical advantages.

Doesn't give fiber

Fiber, a non-absorbable carb that advances gut wellbeing and solid defecations, is just found in plant food varieties. Along these lines, the Carnivore Diet contains no fiber, which may prompt obstruction in certain individuals.

Furthermore, fiber is amazingly significant for the legitimate equilibrium of microscopic organisms in your gut. Truth be told, imperfect gut wellbeing can prompt various issues and may even be connected to debilitated insusceptibility and colon malignant growth. Truth be told, one investigation in 17 men with weight tracked down that a high-protein, low-carb diet essentially diminished their degrees of mixtures that help ensure against colon malignant growth, contrasted with high-protein, moderate-carb diets. By and large, following the Carnivore Diet may hurt your gut wellbeing.

Poor Nutrition Intake

Removing whole nutrition types on any diet can build the danger of supplement inadequacies over the long run. Meat and fish are phenomenal wellsprings of excellent protein and give important sustenance, however they can't give every one of the fundamental nutrients and minerals your body needs to work and flourish appropriately.

Carbs can be found in probably the most supplement thick food varieties on the plant - principally products of the soil. Taking out sugars altogether can likewise dispose of significant wellsprings of key supplements like nutrient C, nutrient A, nutrient E, potassium, and fiber.

Constipation
Fiber is a kind of sugar that assumes a part in sound absorption and assists with keeping things moving. Hence, removing carbs, by and large, may prompt obstruction and GI misery at first.

Increased Heart Health Risks
While greasy fish is a wellspring of heart-solid omega-3s, if a dominant part of your fat admission is coming from other creature-based sources, you're probably going to eat high measures of immersed fat.

Immersed fat, particularly without solid unsaturated fats, is related to expanded blood cholesterol levels and may adversely affect heart wellbeing.

Also, eating a great deal of red meat, particularly handled meats, similar to bacon and hotdog, are related to an expanded danger of coronary illness, diabetes, and disease.

Confused Eating Habits
The more prohibitive your diet, the more it can play with your mental soundness and possibly lead to unfortunate eating practices.

On the off chance that you are finding that keeping away from carbs begins to transform into genuine carb-fear, you should reexamine your methodology.

There is no single food thing - not even carbs - that can represent the moment of truth your wellbeing, and being too exacting with regards to your eating can frequently accomplish more damage than anything else. Also, it makes adhering to your diet long haul almost inconceivable and makes eating way less fun by and large.

May not be appropriate for certain populaces

The Carnivore Diet might be particularly dangerous for specific populaces. For instance, the individuals who need to restrict their protein consumption, incorporating individuals with constant kidney illness, ought not to follow the diet. Likewise, the individuals who are touchier to the cholesterol in food sources, or cholesterol hyper-responders, ought to be mindful about burning-through so some elevated cholesterol food varieties. Besides, certain populaces with uncommon supplement needs would likely not meet them on the Carnivore Diet. This incorporates kids and pregnant or lactating ladies.

Finally, the individuals who have uneasiness about food or battle with prohibitive eating ought not attempt this diet.

What Are the Health Risks of the Carnivore Diet That You Need to Know?

The dangers of the carnivore diet rely upon whether you're following the way to deal with getting in shape or to address an immune system or incendiary condition.

All things considered, "There are a lot of disadvantages to the carnivore diet," says Liz Weinandy, RD, dietitian at The Ohio State University Wexner Medical Center in Columbus. "We have various nutrition classes for an explanation: They each give us a scope of supplements," she says.

Eating just a single nutrition type is an issue, regardless of which one (regardless of whether it's simply vegetables). Restricting yourself to everything meat can make you run low in specific supplements that are bountiful in plants, similar to nutrient C and nutrient E, she says.

Albeit some narrative reports recommend that clogging isn't an issue on a carnivore diet, you are passing up fiber, a supplement significant for colonic wellbeing, says Weinandy. A diet high in red and prepared meats has likewise been connected to an expanded danger of gastric disease, noticed the International Agency for Research on Cancer in an investigation distributed in December 2015 in the diary The Lancet.

(Yet a meta-examination of 42 investigations distributed in May 2017 in the diary Oncotarget revealed that while case-control concentrates on red and handled meat utilization do show this affiliation, partner contemplates — a kind of observational investigation — don't.) Eating a lot of meat protein can likewise put unjustifiable weight on kidneys.

Another thought: Extreme limitation or marking food varieties "great" or "awful" can likewise set off cluttered eating practices or all-out dietary problems, Weinandy says.

Additionally, eating a wealth of foods grown from the ground has been discovered to be connected to expanded joy, life fulfilment, and prosperity.

Reasons the Carnivore Diet Might Still Be Totally Crazy
In the event that you've made it this far into the article, you're likely understanding that the carnivore diet isn't just about as silly as it might from the start sound. In any case, there are some convincing motivations to not attempt it—or if nothing else not follow it for extremely long—aside from what we've effectively referenced.

Environmental Impact
It's protected to say that, if everybody embraced this diet, the world would run out of creatures pretty quick. Supporting natural cultivating practices and eating locally is a respectable, keen approach to improve the government assistance of animals and decrease contaminations, yet radically expanding the interest for meat would without a doubt detrimentally affect the planet—in any event, while ordinary cultivating strategies stay unavoidable.

Vegetables Are Still Good

Carnivore dieters put stomach related issues on plants. Grains, vegetables, and nuts are undoubtedly wellsprings of phytic corrosive, an antinutrient that can forestall the body's retention of iron and zinc. Be that as it may, as per St. Pierre, the adverse consequence it has on your sustenance is insignificant. "The information on phytic corrosive, lectins, and trypsin inhibitors is not even close as terrible as individuals like to describe it," says St. Pierre. Plants have inborn protection frameworks to deter hunters from eating them, however, that doesn't mean they can't or shouldn't be eaten. Likewise, "a lobster has a shell and paws to safeguard itself, however, that doesn't mean you can't eat it," says St. Pierre.

Likewise, the manner in which we plan food decreases the intensity of the antinutrients inside it. At the point when the bread is prepared with yeast, the phytic corrosive substance in the grains scatters. Levels are additionally low in grew grain and sourdough bread. "Simultaneously," says St. Pierre, "insensible sums, phytic corrosive likewise have some potential medical advantages, one of them being against malignant growth, and it can chelate substantial metals." One such weighty metal, iron, can be harmful in high sums. What's more, you hazard getting such sums on an all-meat diet.

It is not necessarily the case that a few groups aren't particularly touchy to certain plant food varieties. On the off chance that you know one that annoys you, don't eat it. In any case, it's most likely best not to get rid of all of the vegetation in your diet depends on a response to a couple of types.

Sustainability

The planet isn't the solitary thing that could endure on the off chance that you go all meat, constantly. You may wind up detesting life, regardless of how cool eating burgers and bacon the entire day sounds to you now. A severe creature diet implies no lager, no avocados for your Fajita Night... and, truth be told, no fajitas by any means (tortillas are a no-no). You can twist the standards and have your cheat days, however then you're not actually doing the diet, right?

Munsey says he didn't get numerous yearnings on the carnivore diet however has since added back certain plants and a periodic carbs for long haul wellbeing. "I still essentially follow the carnivore diet since I love the manner in which I feel on it. Yet, it's truly hard to do when you travel." If you can't discover excellent meat out and about, you should be cautious where you eat out. Yet, that can be important for the excitement of going carnivore, as well.

"It's amusing to arrange two rib-eyes and nothing else and perceive how the server responds," says Munsey. "I was in an air terminal and got four cheeseburger patties and the director came out to affirm that my request was correct. It unquestionably misleads individuals."

Why Are Some Experts So Alarmed About a So-Called 'All-Meat Diet'?

Numerous experts are stressed over the dangers of eating such a lot of soaked fat from meats like greasy steaks and bacon, which is additionally one of the fundamental worries with a keto diet. While the dangers of dietary soaked fat might be discussed, the American Heart Association repeated their position in a position paper distributed in July 2017 in the diary Circulation. The examination, which took a gander at in excess of 100 investigations, noticed that individuals ought to supplant wellsprings of immersed fat with unsaturated fats to bring down the danger of coronary illness.

The World Health Organization (WHO) likewise characterizes a solid diet as one that incorporates natural products, vegetables, vegetables, nuts, and entire grains — all food varieties that are wellsprings of carbs — and zeroing in on unsaturated fats, similar to fish and avocado, while restricting soaked fat from greasy meat and margarine.

There's likewise the possible weight on kidneys while using high measures of protein. You additionally pass up sickness battling supplements, similar to fiber, and cancer prevention agents, similar to nutrient C and E, says Weinandy.

A few groups, who follow this diet, including its makers, highlight clans in history that endure just on specific food varieties. Individuals talk about how the Inuit's ate principally lard and liver, yet, as an article distributed in August 2018 in Popular Science brought up, they additionally eat an assortment of meats, similar to whale skin, which contains nutrient C and a ton of unsaturated fat. This isn't the manner by which carnivore dieters are displaying their food decisions.

Who Should Eat a Carnivore Diet? And Who Shouldn't Eat a Carnivore Diet?

In the event that you trust you have food prejudices, the carnivore diet can fill in as a transient end diet to reveal food varieties that conceivably disagree with your framework. You may attempt this for about a month and a half and afterwards once again introduce new food sources gradually (each likely prejudice in turn) to perceive what does or disagrees with you, says Schmidt.

Be that as it may, in case you're taking a gander at an end diet of any kind, first counsel an enlisted dietitian with information on your wellbeing concerns and clinical foundation. The carnivore diet isn't the best way to do an end diet, says Weinandy. "There is a cycle and convention to distinguish food sources that individuals don't endure. Everybody is unique. We need to take a gander at each person and attempt to devise an arrangement that is ideal for them," she says. Frequently, this can be accomplished by less prohibitive methods.

Regarding who this isn't for, in case you're inclined to confuse about eating, don't go into any diet. What's more, on the off chance that you have an ongoing illness, similar to diabetes or coronary illness, converse with your primary care physician prior to attempting a limited diet like this one. Try not to follow the carnivore diet in the event that you have any degree of kidney infection.

Chapter 3: Benefits of carnivore diet and who should try it.

Creatures with enormous teeth and short stomach related parcels are intended to eat meat. However, shouldn't something be said about individuals? We're omnivores. Is an all-creature diet even workable for us?

As indicated by Brian St. Pierre, R.D., Director of Performance Nutrition at Precision Nutrition, training and counselling organization, plant food sources aren't totally needed in the human diet. "What do we really have to live? We need protein, fat, and nutrients and minerals in specific sums," says St. Pierre. Creature food sources—and meat, explicitly—can apparently cover those requirements (see "Does The Carnivore Diet Create Nutrient Deficiencies?" underneath). That surely doesn't imply that we shouldn't eat plants, in any case, from a sustenance stance, it isn't indispensable that we do, in any event for momentary wellbeing.

The Carnivore Diet for Humans

The thing is, however, besides some segregated ancestral individuals in furthest corners of the world (like the Inuits of cold locales), hardly any individuals have at any point attempted to live on creatures alone. The individuals who have done so essentially on the grounds that no different wellsprings of food were accessible. In any case, the carnivore diet (additionally called a zero-carb diet) has as of late burst into flames. Also, individuals are following it by decision!

Why? For a large number of similar reasons individuals attempt a ketogenic diet: weight loss, more clear reasoning, less stomach related issues, and a straightforward way to deal with eating that allows them to devour food sources they appreciate. It might likewise offer execution benefits. In spite of the fact that rejecting all plant food sources appears to be an extreme advance, it immediately eliminates essentially the entirety of the allergens and antinutrients that a few groups discover mess wellbeing up and distress, and, as with ketogenic diets, the absence of carbs alone can offer a scope of benefits.

With his appearance on the Joe Rogan Experience digital recording in late 2017, and his advancement through the site nequalsmany.com and Instagram, Shawn Baker is the most celebrated defender of the carnivore diet. A muscular specialist and long-lasting medication-free competitor, Baker is in his 50s, torn, and an actual wonder, having as of late set two indoor paddling world records. He professes to have eaten just creature items—restricting him chiefly to rib-eye steaks— for over a year while enduring no chronic sickness impacts and watching his benefits in the rec center take off.

He has a progressing and casual trial, urging any individual who will follow the diet to record his/her involvement in it, however, concedes that he hasn't had his own wellbeing formally assessed since he began eating creatures as it were. Rogan, indeed, recoiled during their meeting when Baker admitted that he hadn't had any blood work done to check where his cholesterol, fatty substances, and aggravation markers evaluated. Luckily, other (human) carnivores have been tried.

Yet, before we talk about the wellbeing impacts of a predatory way of life, we should characterize precisely what it involves.

Why Do People Follow the Carnivore Diet?

You can discover numerous instances of individuals who've shed pounds following the carnivore diet, however as you most likely know, this is essentially a component of energy adjustment and can be accomplished with a diet. At the end of the day, the carnivore diet offers no exceptional weight loss impacts. Numerous individuals just unknowingly eat fewer calories when they can just eat meat, which makes it a lot simpler to get thinner. Much more normal than weight loss brags, notwithstanding, are accounts of individuals utilizing the carnivore diet to relieve or even take out negative side effects they partner with food prejudices or sensitivities.

Food narrow mindedness is an informal term for a reliably negative response to a specific food or nutritional category. For instance, a few group experience negative results, both physical and mental, in the wake of eating wheat, dairy, or matured food sources, and many expect this implies they have a narrow mindedness to something in those food varieties, similar to gluten, lactose, or histamines (which are found in aged food varieties).

You'll likewise regularly hear devotees of the carnivore diet talk about how plants contain "antinutrients," like lectins, phytic corrosive, and gluten, which keep creatures from having the option to process them. These mixtures are without a doubt found in many plant food varieties, including soy, wheat, corn, oats, tomatoes, apples, cherries, potatoes, carrots, zucchini, and others.

Meat doesn't contain any of these mixtures, so by eating only meat, individuals can without much of a stretch stay away from any food sources and substances that may trigger undesirable responses in their bodies. This is sensible. It's fundamentally the initial step of a disposal diet, a logically approved approach to figure out which food varieties you can easily eat and which you can't.

By first eliminating every one of the conceivably dangerous food varieties and afterwards slowly once again introducing them into your diet individually, you can segregate which food varieties you shouldn't eat dependent on how your body reacts to each "challenge". Where the carnivore diet goes a little crazy, nonetheless, is that it never advances past that initial step of the discount end. Rather than utilizing it as a way back to a nutritious, adjusted diet—an unfortunate obligation—numerous individuals consider it to be an objective all by itself.

Does the carnivore diet have health benefits?

The primary thing you need to ask yourself is the thing that your objectives are for this method of eating, and what accommodates your way of life. For the motivations behind this article, I'll partition the carnivore diet into 5 distinct tiers. In light of your objectives, you can choose which tier is ideal for you. I talk about this in significantly more detail in my impending book, "The Carnivore Code: Unlocking the Secrets to Optimal Health by Returning to Our Ancestral Diet."

One other thought in the conversation of what to eat on a carnivore diet is WHEN to eat. I'll do an entirely separate blog entry about discontinuous fasting and time-confined eating. Here's the abbreviated form: in light of the fact that a carnivore diet is so satisfying, the vast majority find that eating two times each day, or even once each day (known as OMAD) works better compared to three suppers each day. This additionally makes time-confined eating a lot simpler by taking into consideration a more compacted eating window with fewer dinners. In the feast designs that follow, I have proposed breakfast, lunch, and supper dinners, however twice or once each day eating is thoroughly proper, and maybe far superior!

Promoters of the carnivore diet guarantee that it has various medical advantages and advances the body's regular capacities.

Its advocates guarantee that it can improve:

- Body weight
- Depression
- Anxiety
- Diabetes
- Skin complaints
- Pain
- Digestive issues
- Arthritis

Since the Carnivore Diet prohibits carbs, it wipes out treats, cakes, sweets, soft drinks, cakes, and comparative high-carb food sources. These food varieties are low in gainful supplements and frequently high in calories. Consequently, they ought to be restricted to a solid, adjusted diet.

High-sugar food sources can likewise be dangerous for individuals with diabetes, as they can spike glucose tiers. Truth is told, restricting refined carbs and sweet food sources are frequently prescribed to control diabetes.

Nonetheless, the total disposal of carbs on the Carnivore Diet hasn't suggested or fundamental for diabetes the executives. All things being equal, eating more modest measures of healthy, high-fiber carbs that don't cause spikes in glucose is suggested.

1. Weight Loss

On an all-meat diet? The vast majority's first response is that you'd get fat, yet that is profoundly improbable. Similarly as with the ketogenic diet, neglecting to take in carbs keeps your glucose low consistently. You don't get insulin spikes, so your body has no motivation to store approaching calories as muscle to fat ratio. Moreover, the restrictions on what you can eat make it practically difficult to get a calorie surplus without a coordinated exertion.

Ryan Munsey, a presentation mentor with a degree in food science and human nourishment, has been on a ketogenic diet for quite a long time. The previous fall, he explored different avenues regarding the carnivore diet for 35 days. "I wasn't attempting to get more fit," he says, "yet I went from 188 to 183 pounds in the main week." Despite the weight loss and the seriously limited food list, Munsey says he never felt even a little bit hungry—most likely in light of the fact that protein and fat are profoundly satisfying supplements. To return weight on, Munsey found that he needed to teach himself to eat two to four pounds of meat every day. "It didn't care for I was stuffing myself, yet it felt bizarre from the outset to eat such a lot of meat."

In case you're the sort who missing mindedly grubs on nuts, pretzels, or other nibble food sources, taking in many calories without seeing, the carnivore diet can help hold you in line. "You must be genuinely eager to eat," says Munsey. It could be not difficult to toss small bunches of popcorn down your neck, yet you can't inadvertently eat a burger or cook a steak. You'll start eating just when you need to and taking in barely enough to keep you fulfilled. "You gain proficiency with the distinction between physiological craving and careless eating," says Munsey.

Likewise, however, it wasn't his objective; Munsey's body remained in a low degree of ketosis all through the five-week diet (he tried ketone tiers to know without a doubt). "A great many people in the keto camp would say in the event that you eat in excess of a pound of meat daily you're not going to be in ketosis," says Munsey. "Yet, I ate as much as four pounds per day and I was."

Will the Meal Plan Help With Weight Loss?

It may. You're eating only one kind of food — meat — so your calories will probably be more limited. For one, there's the satiety that this protein gives. At that point, there's the way that it kills careless eating, says Schmidt. "You don't carelessly eat chicken bosoms. It's an entirely tasteful diet, yet you don't lick your plate," she says.

You may likewise go into a condition of ketosis on the carnivore diet, says Schmidt. Around there, your body is consuming fat for fuel as opposed to carbs. That is not an assurance, however. It's a misguided judgment that all you need is as far as possible carbs to get to ketosis — protein matters, as well.

"In overabundance, protein can prompt an expansion in glucose and insulin tiers, and it can show you out of ketosis," says Schmidt. Know your objectives. In the event that you will likely eat zero carbs, have simply meat. On the off chance that it's to be in ketosis, ensure that you centre predominantly around fattier wellsprings of meat, just as eggs and other fat sources, similar to cheddar and spread.

What Are the Health Risks of the Carnivore Diet That You Need to Know?

The dangers of the carnivore diet rely upon whether you're following the way to deal with get more fit or to address an immune system or incendiary condition.

All things considered, "There are a ton of drawbacks to the carnivore diet," says Liz Weinandy, RD, dietitian at The Ohio State University Wexner Medical Center in Columbus. "We have numerous nutrition types for an explanation: They each furnish us with a scope of supplements," she says.

Eating just a single nutrition type is an issue, regardless of which one (regardless of whether it's simply vegetables). Restricting yourself to everything meat can make you run low in specific supplements that are bountiful in plants, similar to nutrient C and nutrient E, she says.

Albeit some narrative reports propose that blockage isn't an issue on a carnivore diet, you are passing up fiber, a supplement significant for colonic wellbeing, says Weinandy. A diet high in red and prepared meats has additionally been connected to an expanded danger of gastric malignancy, noticed the International Agency for Research on Cancer in an investigation distributed in December 2015 in the diary The Lancet. (However a meta-examination of 42 investigations distributed in May 2017 in the diary Oncotarget detailed that while case-control concentrates on red and handled meat utilization do show this affiliation, partner considers — a sort of observational examination — don't.) Eating a lot of meat protein can likewise put unnecessary weight on kidneys.

Another thought: Extreme limitation or naming food varieties "great" or "awful" can likewise set off cluttered eating practices or all-out dietary problems, Weinandy says.

Also, eating a wealth of leafy foods has been discovered to be connected to expanded joy, life fulfilment, and prosperity.

2. Better Heart Health

Most importantly, as we clarified with all due respect to coconut oil the previous summer, there's still no reasonable connection between the utilization of soaked fat and coronary illness. There is likewise a strong heap of proof that soaked fat can conceivably improve heart wellbeing. Munsey himself discovered that to be the situation.

A couple of months prior to beginning his carnivore diet test, Munsey's blood work uncovered that his complete cholesterol was 180mg/dL, his HDL tier (often called the "great" cholesterol) was 57, and his LDL was 123. Every great score. Following 35 days of carnivore dieting, he had his numbers checked once more.

His absolute cholesterol moved to 241mg/dL. While numerous specialists believe anything more than 200 to be excessively high, some portion of the explanation was the expansion in his HDL—it went up 10 focuses. His LDL went to 162, however his VLDL tiers—considered a significant marker for coronary illness hazard—were estimated at 12, which is very low.

The Mayo Clinic says your cholesterol proportion is a preferable danger indicator over absolute cholesterol or LDL. To discover it, you partition your complete cholesterol number by your HDL score. That gives Munsey a proportion of 3.6 to 1. As 3.4 is viewed as ideal, he's in a sound reach.

Something else about cholesterol: despite the fact that higher LDL numbers are viewed as hazardous, the sort of LDL particles you have moving through your supply routes is generally significant. In the event that they're little and thick, they're viewed as more perilous than if they're greater and "fluffier." Therefore, two individuals with a similar LDL worth could be totally different degrees of hazard.

As per the Cooper Institute, a decent method to figure out what sort of LDL particles you have is to discover your proportion of fatty oils to HDL cholesterol. The lower the proportion, the less the danger. Munsey's fatty substances came in at 59mg/dL, making his fatty substance to-HDL proportion under 1, which is excellent.

Obviously, Munsey followed the diet for a brief timeframe, so it's difficult to anticipate what might befall his body long haul; however it should facilitate your apprehensions about the threats of meat for the cardiovascular framework. Five weeks of eating cow parts didn't give him a coronary episode. Truth be told, it appeared to decrease his odds of having one.

In the event that you don't trust us or Munsey see his authority blood lab, direct from his PCP, beneath.

3. Lower Inflammation

As indicated by certain vegetarians, fat-rich creature food sources elevate aggravation to some extent that is comparable to smoking cigarettes. The reality, in any case, is that they can really bring down it. A recent report in the diary Metabolism thought about subjects who ate a high-fat, low-carb diet to those after a low-fat, high-carb diet. Calories were limited in the two gatherings, yet the high-fat eaters had lower markers of fundamental irritation following 12 weeks. Therefore, the analysts reasoned that high-fat eating might be more advantageous to cardiovascular wellbeing.

The liver produces C-receptive proteins because of irritation, so estimating CRP tiers can show how much aggravation is in your framework. A degree of 10mg/L or less is typical, and 1mg/L or less is acceptable. Munsey's CRP score post-diet was extraordinarily low: 0.34.

Essentially cutting plant food sources from your menu can bring down aggravation without anyone else. "On the off chance that you had a food affectability to a portion of the plants you were eating and had second rate aggravation," says Brian St. Pierre of Precision Nutrition, "at that point eliminating them will cause you to feel much improved."

Lower aggravation can mean fewer throbbing joints. Additionally: "There's some proof that eating more coagulated proteins, as you find in bone stock, collagen, and gelatin," says St. Pierre, "can improve ligament wellbeing." This is examined further in our manual for bone stock.

4. Higher Testosterone

Diets high in fat have been appeared to help testosterone tiers. Indeed, an examination in the American Journal of Clinical Nutrition found that men who followed a high-fat, low-fiber diet for 10 weeks had 13% higher absolute testosterone than subjects who ate low fat and high fiber. It's nothing unexpected then that Munsey's absolute testosterone tiers jumped from 495 ng/dL to 569. Not awful for age 33. "I was setting up a shelter first thing each day," he says.

5. Less Digestive Problems

We've been advised that it is so imperative to eat fiber our entire lives, and have been offered everything from grain biscuits to Metamucil to ensure we get enough. Be that as it may, carnivore dieters believe it's more difficult than it's worth, and science may demonstrate them right.

A recent report in the World Journal of Gastroenterology explored the impacts of lessening fiber consumption in individuals with ongoing clogging—the direct inverse of what most specialists would suggest. Subjects were advised to devour no fiber at all for about fourteen days. At that point, they were permitted to build their fiber admission to a tier they were OK with, or follow a high-fiber diet. Extraordinarily, the vast majority of the subjects were doing great to such an extent that they picked to proceed on the zero-fiber plan. The investigation endured a half year.

The individuals who ate high fiber detailed no adjustment of their condition, however, the individuals who ate no or limited quantities of fiber noted huge upgrades in their indications—including decreased gas, swelling, and stressing. Besides, the ones on zero fiber really expanded the recurrence of their solid discharges!

The explanation fiber-filled eating could be tricky for the gut isn't clear, yet carnivore dieters fault certain mixtures in plant food sources as the wellspring of stomach related problems. They refer to the book The Plant Paradox, by Steven R. Gundry, M.D., which contends that the common safeguard components that plants contain to prevent hunters cause swelling, gas, and other stomach related misery that may make them not worth eating for people. Lectins, gluten, and phytic corrosive—regular in natural products, greens, beans, grains, nuts, and seeds—can add to irritation and auto-insusceptible issues like IBS, Leaky Gut, and the sky is the limit from there. While this is a dubious assessment, it gives clarification as to why carnivore dieters guarantee to feel better compared to they did eating plants.

"We've been told for such a long time that you need this fiber," says Munsey. "Be that as it may, possibly you don't. Perhaps you needn't bother with any. The carnivore diet difficulties what we think we know."

6. Expanded Mental Clarity

Similarly likewise with the ketogenic diet, carnivore dieters report thinking all the more obviously and having better concentrate practically immediately. Once more, similarly as with going keto, there is a break-in period where your body needs to sort out some way to fuel your framework without carbs, so you'll presumably feel dormant and touchy from the outset. You may experience issues resting and even grow awful breath; however, you can brave it. Inside a couple of days or a little more than seven days, you could feel keener than at any other time. Maybe surprisingly better than if you were doing a standard ketogenic diet. "Constantly week, your framework comes on the web," says Munsey.

7. Improved Health

With regards to in general wellbeing and overseeing constant illness, there are some fascinating investigations taking a gander at the potential advantages of keto and other low carb diets on overseeing glucose and diabetes. Yet, once more, these advantages are likely the aftereffect of improved sustenance generally - wiping out added sugar and void calories, while supplanting them with nutritious, entire food varieties.

As a result of the kinds of food advanced on a carnivore diet (high-fat creature items) and the absence of supplement thick plant choices, it is probably not going to give satisfactory, adjusted nourishment and may really hurt wellbeing more than it makes a difference.

To the extent we know there is no logical proof to help taking out all starches from your diet, and we don't perceive any additional medical advantages in doing as such.

8. More straightforward Dieting

There's one thing about the carnivore diet that nobody can contend: it's not confounded. You eat creature food varieties when you're eager, and that is it. In case you're the sort of individual who gets confounded tallying calories or macros, is worn out on gauging parcels on a food scale, or isn't sure what's without gluten and what isn't, a carnivore diet will everything except alleviate you of reasoning.

"I began by attempting to eat one rib-eye in the first part of the day and one PM, or the same measure of protein and fat," says Munsey. "It worked out to be about a pound of meat toward the beginning of the day and afterwards two PM. estimated nothing or followed proportions." It's additionally significant that Munsey likes to follow an irregular fasting way of eating, having his first feast between 10 a.m. furthermore, 12 p.m. what's more, his second somewhere in the range of 3 and 5 p.m. Yet, you don't need to.

"To the extent, your way of life goes, it's very pleasant," says Munsey. "You will eat steak and bacon the entire day. I never became wary of eating meat. I really began desiring it."

And keeping in mind that a meat-rich diet may seem like it would use up every last cent, the sums you really devour may not be high, since meat is so satisfying. That should minimize expenses—particularly in the event that you in a real sense aren't accepting some other food.

Proposed Health Benefits of the Carnivore Diet

A carnivore diet has been acquiring steam as a likely mitigating diet for individuals with immune system conditions, especially considering a portion of the press the diet's gotten. The girl of the way of life master Jordan Peterson, Mikhail, was profiled in August 2018 in the U.K. distribution of The Times, discussing how her diet of meat, salt, and water allegedly alleviated her of her downturn indications.

"This is the most limited end kind of diet. It eliminates any food sensitivities individuals may respond to," says Schmidt. All things considered, the prevalence of the carnivore diet has spread to be a more broad weight loss diet.

Note that this diet is new to the point that there's no exploration on the wellbeing impacts of an all-meat diet if a carnivore diet can really lessen indications of immune system conditions, or in the event that it is a solid strategy for uncovering food prejudices or supporting weight loss.

The Carnivore Diet for Athletes

The ketogenic diet has taken a ton of warmth from pundits who say that individuals who exercise should eat carbs to supply fuel, yet science has shown that in addition to the fact that it is feasible to work out on a low-carb diet, you can even perform at a world-class tier. Yet, remove ALL carbs and all plant food sources and it very well may be an altogether different story. The short answer is that we don't realize precisely what a drawn-out carnivore diet would mean for bulk, perseverance, or generally execution yet. However, numerous carnivore dieters report making probably the best gains of their lives on the arrangement.

As referenced above, Shawn Baker is an elite indoor paddling contender and deadlifts 700 or more pounds at more than 50 years of age. He could well be a hereditary anomaly, yet shouldn't something be said about Ryan Munsey? Without adding bodyweight, Munsey made emotional strength gains on the diet. The following are the upgrades he made on his two-rep max in the different lifts he tried. All were cultivated inside five weeks of carnivore eating.

The primary week on the diet, Munsey says he felt languid and had little inspiration to prepare. In any case, continuously week, he says, he was a "samurai" in the exercise center. He attributes the additions to the expanded measure of protein he was eating, as he had been doing a ketogenic diet earlier. "With keto, I felt extraordinary intellectually, yet I never wanted to do much actually. On the carnivore diet, I just felt like a hero." He was getting 120 to 150 grams of protein each prior day when he weighed somewhere in the range of 185 and 188 pounds. In the wake of embracing a two-to-four-pound each day meat propensity, Munsey gauges his protein admission was somewhere in the range of 200 and 300 grams.

It's significant that Munsey didn't do cardio, aside from day by day strolls (he arrived at the midpoint of 5,000 stages per day, absolute). Accordingly, it's hard to say how he would have fared had he been running, paddling, or accomplishing all the more metabolically requesting exercises like CrossFit. "I think the variation time frame before you would dominate again at those exercises would be more severe than what I went through," says Munsey.

To be reasonable, Baker claims he required a half year to completely adjust to the diet and get his exhibition in the groove again.

"Since we can live on a carnivore diet," says St. Pierre, "doesn't mean we'd fundamentally flourish with it. In case you're a discontinuous game competitor, contending in running or something different that requires high yield for 60–120 seconds, it would be trying to perform well when you're not eating any carbs. There are individuals who receive truly well to fat and their exhibition improves, yet I figure execution would languish over most." As with any diet, you'll need to attempt it and see what occurs.

In the event that you are a competitor or rec centre rodent, you may improve to alter the carnivore diet similarly as we talked about adjusting the ketogenic diet HERE. St. Pierre recommends beginning by adding a few vegetables. "Cruciferous ones like broccoli, cauliflower, and kale would be my vote." If you find that your exercises are enduring, "possibly that implies having an intermittent yam or apple," says St. Pierre.

Will the carnivore diet benefit my performance?

Its defenders guarantee the carnivore diet has assisted with weight loss and mental lucidity. In any case, at this stage, the carnivore diet is definitely not a well-informed diet. There are no exploration concentrates as of now distributed on the wellbeing, security or advantages of the diet, just tales and contextual analyses that are not the most significant level of proof in nourishment research. We do know from these contextual analyses that it very well may be an advantageous diet for certain individuals, yet in addition that it probably won't be the correct diet alternative for other people.

We additionally don't have a clue about the impacts of following the diet long haul. What we DO know from sustenance research, in any case, is that a changed diet that incorporates food varieties from the entire grains, organic product, vegetables, nuts and seeds nutritional categories can be advantageous for our wellbeing and execution.

The Mediterranean diet, for instance, incorporates these nutrition types, a lot of assortment and it's been connected with improved wellbeing results. Most importantly we couldn't actually say whether the carnivore diet is useful for execution and wellbeing, yet we do realize that other dietary examples are. Putting our science cap on, we can see that there is certifiably not a reasonable advantage in picking this dietary example contrasted with different diets that are more changed in food decisions. It's consistently imperative to look for individualized guidance with regards to your diet decisions for execution, as everybody is extraordinary, so there is nothing of the sort as a set in stone diet!

Is a Carnivore Diet Right for You?

There is no current examination to help a carnivore diet as an important instrument for improving wellbeing or advancing weight loss.

On the off chance that you are hoping to get in shape calorie control actually remains your best methodology.

On the off chance that you need to improve your wellbeing, following an essential smart dieting approach is your smartest option.

Examination keeps on recommending that a reasonable, supplement thick diet (counting some carbs) as per a sound way of life, is perhaps the best ways to deal with overseeing and lessening your danger of persistent infection.

You don't have to go to limits to get more fit and improve your dietary patterns. Periodically everything necessary is little changes to see intense enhancements in your prosperity.

So as opposed to redesigning your way of life and attempting the following new diet pattern, attempt the accompanying.

Track your daily food consumption in a sustenance application to become familiar with your definite calorie and large scale objectives and see where you are missing the mark. You may be amazed how your everyday decisions are aiding or harming your advancement.

Discover nutritious alternatives you appreciate eating and add a greater amount of them to your day. This incorporates heaps of supplement thick entire food varieties like natural products, vegetables, and entire grains. You may be finding that zeroing in on eating more nutritious food sources implies you consequently have less space for all the other things.

Zero in on absolute wellbeing from the back to front. This incorporates being thoughtful to yourself and realizing what your body needs to flourish. Diet is just a single piece of the riddle, you'll additionally need to investigate your actual wellness, mentality, rest, feeling, and feelings of anxiety, to give some examples of things.

Make eating better significantly simpler with partition controlled, nutritious dinners prepared and conveyed to your entryway. No more diet disappointment, no more reasons, and not any more anguish. Get RD endorsed menus sponsored by science and worked for results.

The carnivore diet includes eating only creature items (generally meat), water, and salt. As you can figure, this hyper prohibitive methodology can assist individuals with getting in shape (by normally lessening calorie consumption) and can make for a decent initial phase in an end diet, however that is the place where the advantages end. Thus, in the last examination, the carnivore diet is only a more limit adaptation of each and every other low-carb diet out there.

A Final Word on the Carnivore Diet: Should You Try It?

While this diet may sound insane to certain individuals, "as a dietitian, I attempt to be pretty much as receptive as could really be expected. On the off chance that there's an intercession that is working for individuals, I don't limit that," says Rodgers. All things considered, outrageous diets like the carnivore diet acquire a savage after, and a few groups may even permit it to turn into their character. Similarly as with any diet, "it's OK to explore different avenues regarding getting your nourishment, yet ensure it doesn't hurt you. Be sensible about your wellbeing and if your wellbeing is enduring, it's an ideal opportunity to take a gander at another arrangement," she says.

Since it's a trend doesn't mean you need to attempt it — or that it's the panacea of wellbeing as some case. "Temporarily, a carnivore diet most likely will not damage anybody. However, it's a prevailing fashion diet," says Weinandy.

Likewise with most trend diets, it burst onto the scene through major media characters and consideration, not logical exploration or approval. Furthermore, presently it will run its course and catch a lot of consideration and dollars. What you need to know, however, is except if you have genuine stomach related problems and need to follow a disposal diet, the carnivore diet has nothing to bring to the table you. In the event that all you need to do is lose fat, form muscle, get sound, and really make the most of your diet, let me acquaint you with something better.

Conclusion:

The Carnivore Diet is incredibly prohibitive, comprising altogether of meat, fish, eggs, and limited quantities of low-lactose dairy. It's said to help weight loss and a few medical problems; however, no exploration backs these cases.

Furthermore, it's high in fat and sodium, contains no fiber or beneficial plant compounds, and is hard to keep up long haul.

While this diet may sound insane to specific individuals, "as a dietitian, I attempt to be just about as receptive as could really be expected. On the off chance that there's an intercession that is working for individuals, I don't limit that," says Rodgers. Outrageous diets like the carnivore diet acquire a wild after, and a few groups may even allow it to turn into their character. Similarly, as with any diet, "it's all right to explore different avenues regarding getting your nourishment, however, ensure it doesn't hurt you. Be reasonable about your wellbeing and if your wellbeing is enduring, it's an ideal opportunity to take a gander at another arrangement," she says.

Since it's a prevailing fashion doesn't mean you need to attempt it — or that it's the panacea of wellbeing in some case. "Temporarily, a carnivore diet most likely will not damage anybody. Yet, it's a craze diet," says Weinandy.

The planet isn't the solitary thing that could endure if you go all meat, constantly. You may wind up detesting life, regardless of how fabulous eating burgers and bacon throughout the day sounds to you now. An exacting creature diet implies no lager, no avocados for your Fajita Night... and no fajitas by any stretch of the imagination (tortillas are a no-no). You can twist the standards and have your cheat days, yet you're not doing the diet.

Munsey says he didn't get numerous desires on the carnivore diet however certain plants have since added back and intermittent carbs for long haul wellbeing. "I still practically follow the carnivore diet since I love the manner in which I feel on it. Be that as it may, it's truly hard to do when you travel." If you can't discover excellent meat out and about, you should be cautious where you eat out. In any case, that can be important for the excitement of going carnivore, as well.

"It's amusing to arrange two rib-eyes and nothing else and perceive how the server responds," says Munsey. "I was in an air terminal and got four cheeseburger patties and the director came out to affirm that my request was correct. It unquestionably misleads individuals."